D0639041

Contents

✳ PART II ✳
who needs sun protection?

✳ PART III ✳
protecting yourself

foreword

Most Americans are unaware that skin cancer is being diagnosed in epidemic numbers; that within ten years, melanoma may be diagnosed more often than lung cancer within certain segments of the population; and that the cost to the American medical system could be in the tens of billions of dollars.

This epidemic can be slowed through the understanding of individual risk factors, early and continued protection from the sun's ultraviolet rays, and early detection and treatment of the disease. In Australia, educating people in these three areas has resulted in a statistical slowing of a similar epidemic. In the United States, a comparable result can likewise be achieved if public education is undertaken with equal determination.

The Skin Cancer Foundation has led the way in this effort by providing educational material on the Internet and throughout the country. In addition, the American Academy of Dermatology supplies comprehensive material to dermatologists and their patients and helps set up skin cancer screenings each year. The U.S. Environmental Protection Agency and the National Weather Service publish a UV index each day in order to alert the public to use adequate protection. Smaller organizations, such as the Billy Foundation and the Melanoma International Foundation, have also sounded the alarm about the risks associated with overexposure to the sun, but in a country the size of the United States, this list is still too small and unfortunately the message too diluted.

As was done in Australia, the U.S. government—with the backing of the media—should begin a concerted nationwide campaign to educate the American public about methods of skin cancer prevention and detection. The organizations and foundations mentioned above, along with the many others mentioned in this book, should be enlisted to work with state and local governments to help create and implement educational programs in schools, doctors' offices, and anywhere else adults and children can be taught appropriate sun protection methods.

Until such a campaign can be launched, this book will fill the gap. It is intended for parents, teachers, outdoor workers, senior citizens, baby boomers, and anyone else interested in learning the best methods for establishing lifelong habits of sun protection. This book discusses important studies from around the world regarding the incidence of skin cancer. Each chapter has been reviewed by an expert. The message is clear: unprotected exposure to the sun may cause skin cancers, including melanoma. Early and continued sun protection by those at risk, combined with early skin cancer detection and treatment, is the only effective means for combating this potentially deadly disease. This book will arm you with the information you need to effectively protect yourself and your family from the problems associated with sun exposure.

—Albert Rosenthal, MD
Clinical professor of dermatology,
Hahnemann Medical College

acknowledgments

We would especially like to thank Albert Rosenthal, MD, clinical professor of dermatology at Hahnemann Medical College in Philadelphia, for his encouragement and advice. A dedicated dermatologist for several decades, Dr. Rosenthal has seen the devastation caused by skin cancers and is firm in his belief that immediate and constant education is needed to help slow this epidemic.

We would also like to thank Irv and Marilyn Kilstofte for bravely sharing the details of their daughter, Kari Steinke's, tragic fight with melanoma, and for voicing their sense of urgency that more information about this deadly disease be made available to the American public.

Many others have helped to ensure the book is both comprehensive and informative: Jeff Ashley, MD, director of Sun Safety for Kids in Burbank, California; Tony Fransway, MD, of Associates in Dermatology in Fort Myers, Florida, and assistant professor of dermatology at University of South Florida; Peter Gies, Ph.D., senior research scientist at the Australian Radiation Protection and Nuclear Safety Agency in Melbourne; Nancy Krywonis, MD, FRCPC, of Metropolitan Dermatology in Minneapolis; Rhondi Meiusi, MD, of the Edina Eye Clinic in Minneapolis; Madhukar A. Pathak, MB, MS, Ph.D., dermatology research professor at Harvard Medical School; David Polsky, MD, Ph.D., assistant professor at the Department of

Dermatology of New York University School of Medicine; Craig Sinclair, director of the Cancer Education Unit of Cancer Council Victoria, chairman of the Cancer Council Australia Skin Cancer Committee, and director of the World Health Organization Collaborating Centre for the Promotion of Sun Protection; Maureen Pauly Utz, MD, of Metropolitan Dermatology in Minneapolis; and Gregory Scott Williams, health and safety manager at the California Department of Fish and Game. We thank them for their generosity of time and expertise.

We would also like to thank Jasmine Melzer and Veronica Barlow at The Skin Cancer Foundation for finding many elusive details, copyeditor Jessica Beebe for her talent and patience, Tom and Fleury Sommers of Sommers & Associates for exceptional ideas and public relations savvy, Lu Daitzchman at Coolibar for graphics and illustrations, Lionel Barrow for his quest to find "footers," Ann Danaher for accommodating numerous last-minute requests, Cindy Eckelberry and Karri Baumann for clearing time so we could meet deadlines, and our close friends Gail Brottman-Kagan and Jon Kagan for their encouragement, for reading the manuscript, for asking questions, and for understanding canceled dinners.

☀ PART I ☀

understanding the problem

understanding the sun and ultraviolet radiation

This entire book is about sun protection. We love the sun—it feels warm and it is comforting. We need it—it provides us with energy, food, and essential vitamins. And we respect it—we know that without the sun, we can't survive. Yet we also need to protect ourselves from its destructive power.

. . . .
Be AWARE of the Dangers of Sun Exposure

Ancient humans understood the need to protect themselves from the sun and paid tribute to what was thought to be a vengeful deity. The Egyptians built the pyramids for the sun god Ra, hoping to win his favor. The Spaniards sacrificed thousands of their youth on an altar each year to ensure the sun would rise every day. Indeed, people in cultures throughout the world believed the sun was a god—Ra, Helios, Apollo—and many went to extremes to keep this powerful god happy.

But those were times when the harm caused by the sun—blindness, skin lesions, dehydration, and death—was attributed to cruel and deliberate divine decisions over which humans had no control. Today, that decision is yours. When you allow yourself to be exposed to harmful ultraviolet radiation, the direct rays of the sun, you invite skin damage, skin cancer, immune suppression, macular degeneration, and cataracts. The increase in the number of diagnosed cases of these problems is directly related to lifestyles and environmental carelessness—ozone depletion and global warming. Given this knowledge, which is backed by decades of scientific studies, you can and should take measures to protect yourself. Be AWARE of the problems associated with sun exposure. Protect yourself and your family by following these steps:

A—avoid unprotected exposure at any time but especially during the hours of peak ultraviolet radiation (between 10:00 A.M. and 4:00 P.M.)

W—wear sun protective clothing, including a long-sleeve shirt, a hat with a three-inch brim, and sunglasses, and seek shade

A—apply broad-spectrum sunscreen with a sun protection factor (SPF) of 30 or higher to all unprotected skin twenty minutes before exposure and reapply every two hours while exposed

R—routinely check your whole body for changes in your skin and report suspicious changes to a physician

E—express the need for sun protection to your family and community

Throughout this book, we use information available from government and private institutions, scientists, and doctors to clarify why and how you can best protect yourself and still enjoy a life filled with activities in the sun. As part of our advice to be AWARE, we strongly

Most dermatologists believe broad-spectrum sunscreens with an SPF of 15 or higher may help prevent melanoma.

advocate that you, your family, your schools, and your local, state, and federal government take a more active role in understanding the need for sun protection, telling others, and providing protection when possible.

To begin, this chapter gives a simplified explanation of how *ultraviolet radiation* (UVR) is measured and how it harms you. The information comes from several sources, including the U.S. Environmental Protection Agency (EPA), the Australian Radiation Protection and Nuclear Safety Agency, The Skin Cancer Foundation, and the American Academy of Dermatology (AAD). Understanding how UVR is harmful is the first and most important step to a lifetime of sun protection.

Ultraviolet Rays Are Harmful

The sun, like all stars, is a huge ball of gases, mostly hydrogen, with about 10 percent helium and other elements. A constant nuclear reaction in the core of the sun changes the hydrogen to helium and then releases tremendous amounts of energy in the form of electromagnetic radiation. Put simplistically, this radiation travels through space in the form of waves. We are actually able to see some of these rays in the form of visible light, but most are invisible to the naked eye. Some, like X-rays, are short and fast, and others, like radio waves, are very long. The entire range of these different wavelengths makes up the electromagnetic spectrum. UVR falls in the middle of this spectrum and includes UVA, UVB, and UVC. UVC is absorbed by the atmosphere and does not reach the earth's surface.

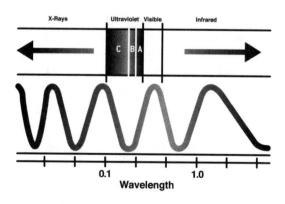

figure 1.1: Electromagnetic Spectrum

Tanning is a serious danger to young people's skin.

However, UVA and UVB are potentially lethal to humans when absorbed by the skin.

How UVR Damages Your Skin

When UVR strikes the skin, it scatters, is reflected, or is absorbed. The UVR that is absorbed causes damage to the cells' *deoxyribonucleic acid* (DNA), which in turn triggers a response, whether it be proliferation, toxic change, mutation, or death. UVA, UVB, and man-made UVC can be absorbed and have an effect at the cellular level. The types of ultraviolet radiation described here are measurements of the sun's rays. Other man-made sources can produce this radiation and are discussed later.

UVC radiation includes wavelengths between 100 and 280 nanometers. These rays are referred to as *germicidal radiation* because they kill microorganisms, including bacteria. UVC is the shortest UVR wavelength and the most intense. As mentioned, it is completely absorbed by the stratosphere, ozone, and atmospheric gases, so the only sources on earth are artificial. Few people are ever exposed to UVC.

UVB radiation includes wavelengths between 280 and 315 nanometers. These rays represent only 2 percent of the sun's energy and are partially absorbed by the ozone layer. Only 15 percent of the UVB entering the atmosphere reaches the earth's surface. Yet even in small amounts, UVB is absorbed by chromosomes and cell proteins and is a major threat to your skin. UVB accounts for most sunburn and the vast majority of skin damage, including premature aging (which we'll discuss in chapter 3) and skin cancers (which we'll discuss in chapters 5 and 6). Your DNA easily absorbs UVB radiation. This changes the shape of the DNA molecule in one of several ways.

UVA radiation includes wavelengths of 315 to 400 nanometers. Of the three types of UVR, UVA has the longest wavelength and is the least powerful. It plays an essential role in the formation of vitamin D, which we'll discuss in chapter 8. However, UVA has been shown to penetrate more deeply than UVB when striking the surface of the skin, harming DNA and compromising the immune system. This in turn destroys your natural defense to cancer. Furthermore,

The incidence of melanoma in the United Kingdom doubled between 1980 and 2000 (Patient UK 2004).

UVA, like UVB, damages your eyes. Depending on the time of year, there can be thirty to fifty times as much UVA as UVB.

Exposure to the combination of UVB and UVA is an attack on the skin. It hits at every level, creating damage that ranges from sunburn to premature aging to malignant melanoma (skin cancer). And for many people, it doesn't take more than twenty minutes for the damage to begin.

Sunburn is the skin's acute and painful response to overexposure to the sun. The skin turns red, becomes tender or swollen, and can blister, then peel. The minimum exposure to UVR required to produce a sunburn varies with each person and is referred to as the MED, or *minimal erythemal dose*. Most white skin (or skin types I, II, and III, which we'll discuss in chapter 7) will burn in less than twenty minutes in the summer or in geographical regions close to the equator. First-degree burns can occur in less than two hours, and skin will blister—reaching second- and possibly third-degree burns—within eight hours. Sunburned cells under a microscope have the same appearance as cancer cells. People with dark skin may not burn, but there is increasing evidence that sun exposure creates similar health problems, including melanoma.

Tanning is a delayed reaction that becomes visible about seventy-two hours after exposure. It is the result of an increased production of melanin, one of the cellular responses to the absorption of UVR. Doctors consider tanning to be evidence of skin damage, and UVB wavelengths are primarily responsible for this damage. While tanning booth operators claim that only "harmless" UVA is used, tanning booths may cause even more serious damage than sun exposure, since UVA penetrates the layers of skin even more deeply than UVB.

Regardless of how they are acquired, sunburns and tans are forms of *phototrauma*, or injury to the skin from overexposure to and absorption of UVR. In May 2000, the National Institutes of Health (NIH) added solar ultraviolet radiation and exposure to sunlamps and tanning beds to the list of identified *carcinogens* (substances known to cause cancer). Two years later, NIH extended this to include broad-spectrum ultraviolet radiation and specifically stated that each component—UVA, UVB, and UVC—was reasonably anticipated to be a human carcinogen.

Skiers get as much UVR on the slopes as on a summer beach.

. . . .

Ozone Thinning Increases UVR Exposure

The *ozone layer* forms a thin shield in the *stratosphere,* a region more than six miles (ten kilometers) above the earth's surface, and is essential to preventing the sun's harmful rays from reaching the earth. *Ozone* is a naturally occurring gas that absorbs UVR. This absorption in turn keeps the ozone balanced.

An imbalance in the ozone layer occurs when too many man-made gases interact with the ozone. During the 1970s, scientists discovered that such an imbalance had occurred, that ozone was being destroyed, and that the ozone layer was being depleted. When the layer of ozone is depleted, increased UVR reaches the earth's surface, which results in overexposure—damaged skin, skin cancer, macular degeneration, and cataracts.

To date, the main cause of ozone depletion has been the production of *chlorofluorocarbons* (CFCs). These were first used widely as refrigerants, insulating foams, and solvents. Later they were used as spray propellants in paints, cleaners, deodorants, hairsprays, and countless other products. CFCs are carried by air currents into the stratosphere, a process that can take as long as five to ten years. Once there, they absorb UVR, break apart, and react with ozone, eventually breaking it down.

The most severe ozone loss was discovered over Antarctica. This thinning is now commonly called the *ozone hole.* Other areas of depletion have included the Arctic and northern middle latitudes. Ozone depletion increases the amount of UVR reaching the earth and makes these areas more hazardous for human life.

Recognizing the danger of a thinning ozone layer to humans and other living creatures, the United States, along with several other countries, has banned the production of CFCs. Furthermore, there are now international control measures aimed at reducing the release of CFCs and other ozone-depleting substances. However, a recovery of the ozone layer is not expected until late in the twenty-first century. Until then, a 1 percent sustained decrease in the ozone layer may result in a 2 percent increase of UVB and a continued increase in diagnosed skin cancers and other sun-related health problems

May is National Melanoma/Skin Cancer Prevention and Detection Month.

(Scotto 1986). These predicted increases in skin problems may be lessened if sun exposure behavior improves.

....

Global Warming Intensifies UVR Exposure

Natural fluctuations in energy emitted by the sun, combined with a growing concentration of certain gases (such as carbon dioxide) in the atmosphere, have caused temperatures on the earth to rise, a condition known as *global warming*. Scientists are only beginning to understand the consequences of this condition. Not only will global warming cause rising sea levels and extreme weather patterns, but the emissions and pollutants within the atmosphere will interact to create gases which in turn affect the ozone. Further depletion of the ozone combined with the reflective properties of these gases will intensify the amount of UVR people receive and ultimately increase the numbers of diagnosed skin cancers.

....

Using the UV Index

The thinning ozone layer and global warming are not, however, the only causes of the epidemic of skin cancer in the United States and in other Western countries. A general lack of awareness that UVR can be harmful has allowed most Americans to adopt a lifestyle without sun protection. By comparison, this cultural behavior is slowly changing in Australia as a result of years of public education, and it can change here.

In an effort to educate people about the amount of UVR they are exposed to daily, the EPA and the National Weather Service provide a daily UV index. The UV index allows you to make informed decisions about what kinds of sun protection methods to use each day. It is the first step toward being AWARE of the times of day UVR is most hazardous and toward choosing appropriate sun protection.

Squamous cell carcinoma often occurs on the legs of older African-American women (SCF 2003a).

What Is the UV Index?

The *UV index* is produced by a computer model that uses multiple variables to determine the next day's maximum UVR level or to forecast peak UV hours. These are the hours when it is most important for you to use effective sun protection or avoid being exposed. The UV index predicts the daily UVR intensity at solar noon on a scale of 0 to 11 plus, ranking the risk from low to extreme. The following variables affect the model's prediction.

Ozone. Areas where the ozone layer has been depleted will have higher amounts of UVA and UVB. The weather, time of year, and latitude all affect the thickness of the ozone layer and UVR intensity.

Elevation. UVR intensity increases in high-altitude areas because there is less atmosphere to absorb the damaging radiation.

Latitude. At the equator, UVR travels the shortest distance, because the sun is almost directly overhead. Also, the ozone layer is thinner in these hot areas, so there is less protection. At higher latitudes (as you move away from the equator), the sun appears lower in the sky and UVR must travel a greater distance through an atmosphere richer in ozone. The further away from the equator, the less UVR.

Time of year. The intensity of UVR varies with the changing seasons. In areas close to the equator, there is little variation, so there are high levels of UVR year-round. In areas away from the equator, UVR intensity is highest during the summer months.

Time of day. The sun is at its highest point at the noon hour. This means ultraviolet rays have the shortest distance to travel through the atmosphere, making radiation the most intense. In the early morning and late afternoon, the intensity of UVB is greatly reduced. UVA levels are not sensitive to ozone and vary throughout the day according to weather.

Spray-on tans do not provide sun protection.

Cloud cover. Cloud cover reduces UVR levels, but not completely. Even on a cool summer day with full cloud cover, exposed skin can burn.

Interpreting the UV index and Taking Action

Once you know what the UV index will be for a given day, you can determine which methods of sun protection to use. During the peak hours of 10:00 A.M. to 4:00 P.M., you should be particularly AWARE of the dangers of unprotected exposure.

UV index values are grouped into exposure categories. As the standards are more widely accepted, you will see these values reported, probably using colors (green, or low, to red, or high). As a general rule, if the index does not include the effects of cloud cover, it will be called a "clear-sky" or "cloud-free" UV index.

The World Health Organization, the World Meteorological Organization, the United Nations Environmental Programme, and the International Commission on Non-Ionizing Radiation Protection have helped create standards for interpretation of this index. We have combined their guidelines to provide the following advice.

UV range less than 2 is low and no protection is required. You can safely stay outside.

UV range 3 to 5 is moderate, which requires protection. Seek shade during midday hours. Wear sun protective clothing, including a hat with a three-inch brim and sunglasses. Apply sunscreen to all exposed skin and reapply every two hours.

UV range 6 to 7 is high, which requires protection. Seek shade during midday hours. Wear sun protective clothing, including a shirt, a hat with a three-inch brim, and sunglasses. Apply sunscreen to all exposed skin and reapply every two hours.

UV range 8 to 10 is very high, which requires extra protection. Avoid being outside during midday hours. Make sure to seek shade. Wear sun

From 1973 to 1999, the incidence of eye melanomas increased 295 percent (SCF 2003c).

protective clothing, including a shirt, a hat with a three-inch brim, and sunglasses. Apply sunscreen to all exposed skin and reapply every two hours.

UV range 11 is extreme and requires caution. Avoid being outside during midday hours. Make sure to seek shade. Wear sun protective clothing, including a shirt, a hat with a three-inch brim, and sunglasses. Apply sunscreen to all exposed skin and reapply every two hours.

Where to Find the UV Index

Many radio and TV weather reports now include the UV index. To help fight the epidemic of skin cancers in this country, all weather reports on every news program should include the UV index and explain what it is, why it is important, and what methods of sun protection are appropriate. In Australia this is done routinely, keeping the general population aware of the harm of exposure and giving suitable advice for protection.

Currently, there are a number of different Internet sources for the UV index in the United States (see "Online Resources" at the back of the book). Local television stations often provide a link from their Internet weather forecasts. Like a daily weather forecast, the UV index provides you with the information you need to make appropriate decisions about sun protection.

. . . .
Indirect UVR Exposure

The UV index does not monitor indirect or reflected UVR. These are rays that "bounce" from surfaces such as sand, concrete, water, snow, and buildings. Indirect UVR adds to the amount of exposure you receive. This is especially important to consider when you are using a hat or shade as a protection method, since indirect UVR can still cause burns. Further, UVA—unlike UVB—does pass through glass.

There is a huge amount of misinformation about
skin cancer on the Internet.

So always assume that you will be exposed to some level of indirect UVR and use combined methods of sun protection accordingly.

· · · · · · · · · · · · · · · ·
Artificial UVR

There are many different instruments or machines that can expose us to UVR. Most that are found in the workplace have industry standards and regulations that provide protection when those standards are enforced. However, the most common machine that exposes people to UVR, causing premature aging and skin cancers, is the tanning bed.

Tanning beds subject users to large amounts of UVA and generally lesser amounts of UVB. Our own 2003 survey of dermatologists at the annual meeting of the AAD suggests that many believe tanning booths should be banned because they contribute to the skin cancer epidemic. Some states now have laws against their use by children.

Summing Up

The sun's powerful rays affect you both positively and negatively. Our planet depends on these rays, yet premature aging and skin cancers are a common consequence of too much exposure. Exposure to UVA and UVB alters the DNA structure in your cells, which can cause irreversible damage. Protection from these rays is the only way to avoid these problems. You can use the UV index to find out tomorrow's predicted peak UVR level and be AWARE of effective methods of protection.

Nonmelanoma skin cancers are a costly burden to the medical system.

tanning trends in the United States

In this chapter, we'll take a look at the rise and fall of tanning as a fashion trend. You will see how tanning has been a reflection of changing ideas about appropriate behavior and clothing for women, and how a growing awareness of the risks of sun exposure will ultimately end this trend.

. . . .

The Nineteenth Century: From Sunbonnets to Swimsuits

In the nineteenth century, wealthy Americans worked hard to establish their social status by copying their counterparts in Europe. Tans were considered boorish and lower class. "Ladies" were especially careful to avoid exposure to the sun and took great pains to keep their skin flawless. This indicated both their class and their wealth. In the Southern states, for example, where the only property women owned was their clothes, ladies' clothing was made from the most expensive materials from around the world, and they never left the house without elaborate sunbonnets and gloves to protect their skin. The paler you were and the more elaborately you dressed, the richer you appeared.

By the mid-1800s, however, swimming had become an acceptable recreation for both men and women. Beach vacations were more accessible, as there was a growing network of train lines and a growing middle class. Consequently, the evolution of bathing suits accelerated. Women were not encouraged to swim, but bloomers covered only by skirts with knee socks became part of their beach ensemble.

It was only at the end of the nineteenth century that swimming was finally recognized as a sport for both men and women. Along with this recognition came tailored bathing suits for women that allowed for better movement in the water. These suits seem modest by today's standards, but they were the beginning of a trend to expose more skin to the sun.

Tans, however, were still not fashionable. Beachgoers continued to protect their skin by wearing cover-ups and sitting under houselike canvas structures and umbrellas.

Swimming suits for women would continue to get smaller, more practical, and more revealing as the nineteenth century came to a close. Then, in 1909, Australian Annette Kellerman was arrested for wearing a loose-fitting one-piece suit that barely covered the tops of her legs. Pictures of her in the suit appeared around the world, and one year later, this type of suit was the norm. Skin exposure became part of vacation culture, and the problems associated with this exposure began to increase.

· ·

The 1900s through 1960s: Tanning Becomes Fashionable

At the beginning of the twentieth century, bathing suits were small, vacations at beach resorts were fashionable, and tanning seemed inevitable. In the 1920s, Gabrielle "Coco" Chanel, who was famous for her *maison de couture* and beautifully tailored suits for women, returned from a vacation on the French Riviera with a tan. Fashion headlines around the world carried the story, and by the following summer, tans

Brown-eyed people proved 80 percent more
likely to develop cataracts (SCF 2002).

were a symbol of social status. The tide had turned; tanning was now fashionable.

Swimsuits changed even more dramatically in the 1930s and 1940s and came to resemble what they are today. Curiously, this resulted not from fashion trends but from wartime rationing. In 1945 the U.S. government ordered a 10 percent reduction in fabric used in women's swimwear. The skirt and front panel disappeared. In the same year, Louis Reard made further reductions by designing the bikini (named after the Bikini Islands, where a nuclear device had been exploded). While first seen as immodest, the bikini continues to be the preferred style for young women, allowing for more exposure to UVR than any other designed garment.

The First Tanning Products

While swimsuit styles changed and tans became fashionable, there was nothing to protect pale skin from burning other than common sense. In 1914 pharmacist George Bunting from Baltimore invented Noxzema, originally called "Dr. Bunting Sunburn Remedy." It was applied at the end of the day to soothe itching and dry skin. However, burning, peeling, and freckles were all considered a normal part of the tanning process. In the 1930s, Australian chemist H. A. Milton Blake produced another sunburn cream believed to help relieve the problems associated with burned skin.

It was not until 1936 that Eugene Schueller, the founder of L'Oreal, invented the first sunscreen. At the time, though, there was little interest among the general public in preventing tanning or burning. Interest began to grow, however, as American soldiers stationed in the South Pacific experienced intense and debilitating burning. Benjamin Green, a pharmacist in Miami, recognized the growing demand for something that would enhance tanning rather than burning and began experimenting at home. In 1944 Green created the first Coppertone suntanning cream, using household ingredients and testing his invention on himself. By 1945 the company added suntan oil to its product list and began advertising with the slogan "Don't be a paleface." In less than five years, sales reached almost $4 million (Coppertone 2002). By 1950, baby oil, which had been used primarily

Melanoma vaccines are still experimental and unproven.

for rashes on baby bottoms and as a skin lubricant, had become a necessity for sun worshippers. Johnson and Johnson sales boomed. Three years later, Coppertone introduced the predecessor to the present-day Little Miss Coppertone, which appeared on billboards around Miami. By 1956 the world-famous Little Miss Coppertone icon was created.

By now dark tans—the darker the better—were fashionable for all socioeconomic groups. Whole industries sprang up to help people absorb the sun's rays and enhance their tans. Lotions, metallic reflectors, outdoor lounge chairs, and sun mats all beckoned white America to get tan.

By the 1950s, it was well known that getting sunburned was not good for the skin. Sunburns can be painful and even debilitating, and people understood that it "weathered" or aged the skin. Unfortunately, it would take many more decades before people knew that tanning is also potentially life threatening. Responding to the fashion of tanning, manufacturers introduced sunscreens that promoted a deep tan without burning. People thought they were safe.

With the 1960s came the surfing culture, and cocoa butter, richer and more moisturizing than baby oil, soon became the tanning lotion of choice across the country. The prevailing culture—movies, music, books, and television—all heralded the bronzed surfer, who overnight had come to symbolize a lifestyle of health and glamour. By the 1970s, a year-round tan was highly desirable.

. . . .

The 1970s to the Present: The Fashionable Tan Begins to Fade

During the last thirty years of the twentieth century, the tide began to turn once again. More and more methods were being developed to produce tans, while more and more information was being released about the dangers of tanning.

One of the monumental developments in the tanning industry was the invention of the tanning bed. (We'll discuss tanning beds more fully later in this chapter.) It was in the 1970s that Friedrich Wolff, a German scientist, created this device. At the time, Wolff was

Dilation of the eye when wearing proper sunglasses does not allow passage of UVR (Gies, Roy, and Elliott 1990).

studying the effect of sunlight on athletes. During his studies, he used artificially produced UVR. The tans that resulted from a few short minutes of exposure were clearly something that would be attractive to the general public. This prompted Wolff to refine his original designs so that tanning beds could be sold commercially.

When tanning beds first arrived in the United States, they were used therapeutically by people hoping to relieve symptoms of various skin problems. It was not until the late 1980s that they became a popular tanning method.

In the meantime, the public had grown more concerned about "burning." It had become common knowledge that *burning* could lead to cancers later in life, but there was still little concern about *tanning*. People wanted sunscreen that would allow them to stay in the sun without burning. This was a complete misunderstanding of the need for sunscreen, and when researchers established the first sun protection factor (SPF) system in the United States, people used the numbers as a way of determining how long they could stay outside.

By the end of the 1980s, melanoma was being diagnosed at increasing rates in the United States. In Australia, the surfing and beach capital of the world, it was considered epidemic. The numbers of diagnosed melanomas were so high in Australia that the government began a national campaign against skin cancer. "Slip, Slop, Slap" was introduced—slip on a shirt, slop on sunscreen, slap on a hat.

In the 1990s, more people understood the harmfulness of exposure to UVB, and sunscreen was well established as an important method of sun protection. Dozens of different types of lotions—waterproof, sweatproof, SPF 15, SPF 30, SPF 45, aloe, zinc, PABA free—were launched in an effort to protect skin. Tanning, however, remained a top priority, especially for teenagers and young people.

By 1994 it was generally agreed among dermatologists and researchers that intense and repeated exposure to the sun can cause skin cancer. Little Miss Coppertone covered up for the first time as part of a public education campaign for the launch of the UV index.

Encourage student leaders to wear a hat when outdoors.

The Consequences of Tanning

The fashion of tanning is directly responsible for substantial increases in the rate of diagnosed melanoma in the United States. Within fifteen years of the debut of Coco Chanel's French Riviera tan, doctors began to see a rise in the rates of skin-related illnesses, particularly skin cancers. The lifetime risk of melanoma began to climb sharply by the 1980s (see figure 2.1). While other types of cancer—such as breast, lung, colon, and prostate cancer—are now diagnosed more frequently, when projections are compared, we found the number of newly diagnosed cases of melanoma will surpass lung cancer in white-skinned Americans by the year 2020.

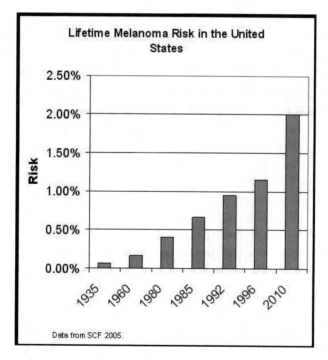

figure 2.1: Lifetime Melanoma Risk in the United States

Good sunglasses can help prevent problems by protecting your eyes.

· · · · · · · · · · · · · · ·

Tanning Beds

Tanning devices have been around since the 1970s, but the tanning salon, complete with a tanning bed, did not become truly popular until about 1990. In the late 1980s, there were fewer than 10,000 businesses that owned tanning beds. By 2000 there were about 50,000 (Pouliot 2003). In 2003 an estimated 29 million Americans visited a tanning salon, compared with 27 million in 2000. By 2004, it was a $5 billion industry and growing (Levine 2004).

Ironically, the rapid expansion of the tanning bed industry was fueled by the growing body of evidence that overexposure to the sun could be deadly. The UVB rays of the sun were thought to be the most damaging, so the tanning industry responded by creating bulbs designed to give off 90 to 95 percent UVA and only 5 to 10 percent UVB. The misperception is that because UVA does not burn, it does no harm.

In fact, UVA rays increase the risk of skin cancer, particularly melanoma (Autier et al. 1994). According to the AAD (2004c), more than 1 million new cases of skin cancer will be diagnosed in the United States in 2004. Many studies suggest that the use of tanning beds contributes to this growing number (Sekula-Gibbs 2004).

UVA is also a strong immune suppressant, helping skin cancers to spread. In May 2000, the National Toxicity Program and the NIH added tanning beds and sunlamps to the list of known carcinogens, yet the number of people using them continues to rise.

Use of Tanning Beds by Youth

While 70 percent of tanning bed users are adult women, female teens between sixteen and nineteen are one of the fastest growing categories of users (Levine 2004). Every year more than 2 million teenagers in the United States visit tanning booths (Dellavalle et al. 2003). These children are convinced tans make them look better but are clearly unaware of the risks. The Cancer Council of New South Wales, Australia (2002), reports that people who use tanning devices

Sunglasses should have standard labels for the percentage
of UVA and UVB blocked.

have two and a half times the risk of squamous cell cancer and one and a half times the risk of basal cell cancer. For those who first used tanning devices under the age of twenty, that increases to over three and a half times the risk for squamous cell cancer. Further, these cancers are showing up in younger and younger people.

Despite the clear correlation between tanning bed use and an increased number of diagnosed skin cancers in younger people, France is the only country out of six—including Australia, Canada, New Zealand, the United Kingdom, and the United States—that bans children from using indoor tanning devices (Dellavalle et al. 2003). In the United Kingdom, suits are being brought against parents and tanning bed operators under child abuse laws to try to curb use by children. In Australia, the Cancer Council of New South Wales has called for amendments to the Public Health Act to closely regulate the tanning bed industry, particularly with regard to protecting children and informing users of risks. Only three American states (Texas, Illinois, and Wisconsin) have laws to keep children from using tanning beds.

If more state legislators understood the harm and the cost tanning beds cause, they would be more likely to address the need for protection.

Misunderstandings and Misperceptions about Tanning Beds

Misunderstandings about the dangers of tanning beds arise from common misperceptions about these devices and from the aggressive marketing by the industry propagating these same misconceptions. Below, we clarify some of the most common misunderstandings or misconceptions about tanning beds.

Getting a base tan from a tanning bed helps protect skin from burning; you should get a base tan before going on vacation. This appears to be the most common myth about possible benefits from indoor tanning. A tan, regardless of how it is acquired, is considered damaged skin and provides an SPF of only 2 to 4 (Pathak 2002).

Cataracts affect most people if they live long enough.

When you consider that most sunscreens offer an SPF of 15, 30, 45, or more, you realize that an SPF of 2 offers little—if any— protection.

Tans acquired slowly are generally healthy and provide protection for the skin. Again, tans only provide an SPF of 2 to 4 (Pathak 2002), and repeated exposure to UVR of any dosage is known to cause skin cancers, including melanoma, wrinkling, and premature aging.

Americans need tanning beds to help produce vitamin D. To the contrary, most Americans get plenty of vitamin D from enriched foods. (We'll discuss vitamin D in more detail in chapter 8.)

Tanning beds relieve depression. To some extent, this may be true. A highly publicized but very small study does indicate that some people find that they feel addicted to the good feeling associated with tanning (Feldman et al. 2004). The theory is that UVR causes the release of *endorphins,* which are nature's way of relaxing you or making you feel better. However, despite this short-term positive feeling, the long-term effect is an increase in the risk of skin cancer and possibly death. If you suffer from *seasonal affective disorder,* a mild depression caused by an absence of light during the winter, your doctor will probably suggest using bright fluorescent light to help relieve symptoms. Do not use a tanning bed for this, because it will only damage your skin.

We hope that as these misconceptions about tanning beds are dispelled, state lawmakers will be more willing to pass legislation protecting citizens from harm. Texas, Illinois, and Wisconsin have led the way. More states will follow as lawmakers and parents begin to understand the potentially life-threatening risks involved in using these devices.

Minimum Precautions for Using Tanning Beds

We strongly recommend that you not use tanning beds. Keep in mind that tans are a symptom of damaged skin and that it logically follows that tanning beds will cause wrinkles, brown age spots,

Sunglasses can help prevent cataracts.

blotching, and leathery, sagging skin that looks older than it is. There is nothing attractive about any of that. If, however, you still use a tanning bed, at the very least follow these precautions:

* Understand the risks involved.

* Do not use a tanning bed if you are under sixteen without permission from your parents or physician.

* Do not use a tanning bed if you burn easily or have fair to olive skin and light to medium hair and eyes.

* Do not use a tanning bed if you already have skin cancer or have a family history of skin cancer.

* Do not use a tanning bed if you are using medication that causes heightened sensitivity to UVR or if you have health problems affected by heat or light.

* Limit your exposure.

* Use goggles to protect your eyes.

Taxing Tanning Salons Could Fund Sun Protection Education

The American Medical Association and the AAD are urging legal action that would ban the sale and use of tanning equipment for nonmedical purposes. Given that this is a $5 billion per year industry, we believe this will be a difficult task. However, if the dangers of tanning beds were viewed as similar to the problems associated with cigarette smoking, placing a tax on the use of tanning beds (like the taxes on cigarettes) could provide the revenue needed for an ongoing national sun protection education campaign. As tanning industry sales are currently at $5 billion yearly, a 2 percent tax for education would provide $100 million annually. If compared to the recommended spending levels in Australia for sun protection education

Employers can play an important role in protecting outdoor workers from UVR exposure.

(Carter, Marks, and Hill 1999), this would adequately cover the ongoing annual costs of a national program for the United States, including the administrative costs of collecting the tax.

. . . .

Fake Tans: The Best Alternative

Despite increasing awareness that tanning is harmful, it is still considered one of the most important elements to looking fashionable. Fortunately, many are wisely looking for alternative ways to gain the glowing shade of tan so highly esteemed. While there are no long-term studies about the effects of fake tans, they appear to be the least dangerous way to change the appearance of skin color. According to market researchers, self-tanners are the fastest growing segment of the sun care market (Mintel Market Researchers 2001).

A Brief History of Fake Tans

Fake tans have been marketed since the 1920s. The Codytan, a self-tanning liquid and powder, appeared in 1929. World War II increased interest in fake tanning with "leg makeup," which helped compensate for a shortage of stockings.

In 1960 Coppertone introduced the first sunless tanning lotion, QT, or Quick Tanning Lotion. This did not wash off; it actually changed the color of skin. While this product was a breakthrough in the tanning industry, uneven application caused orange knees and streaky legs. By 1988, as the damaging effects of sun exposure became better known, several other sunless tanning products appeared on the market in the form of gels, creams, powders, and sprays. These had better results than the earlier products, and by 2002—with the help of Jennifer Lopez—spray-on tanning became the most popular of the fake tan techniques.

In Australia, most employers have sun protection policies.

Spray Tans

You can get a fake tan in just minutes by standing in a booth while a machine sprays you with lotion. Or, you may choose the more labor-intensive method of having someone "paint" you with an airbrush. The tanned appearance from spray tans usually lasts four to six days. Spray tanning salons can be found in hotels, health clubs, malls, and even laundromats across the country. They have become a vital product offered by most tanning salons as an alternative to a UVR tan.

The ingredients for fake tans generally do not include sunscreen. If you use fake tanning products, you should also use sunscreen and other sun protection methods and continue to be AWARE of the problems associated with UVR exposure. If you must have a tan, choose a fake tan rather than expose yourself to UVR. However, we hope you will come to appreciate and protect the beauty of the color you were born with.

Summing Up

The obsession with tanning in this country has contributed to the epidemic of skin cancer we are now experiencing. Sun lotions were originally formulated to block burning and facilitate tanning. Tanning beds were then promoted as a safe way to tan without burning, but instead they have added to the problem. Suntans are a symptom of skin damage. Fake tans are a safer alternative to suntans, although you must still use sun protection methods. Dermatologists and skin specialists around the world would like to see tans go out of fashion.

Seventy-three percent of sunscreen users end up getting sunburned (Wright, Wright, and Wagner 2001).

premature aging of the skin

We all want to look our best as we grow older, so it seems unfair that the skin of the face shows signs of age far sooner than the skin on other parts of the body. Lines, wrinkles, and blotching are common and, despite efforts to the contrary, seem to be appearing at earlier ages. There are, however, ways to slow down the aging process once you understand why it happens.

There are two types of aging, intrinsic and extrinsic. *Intrinsic,* or internal, aging is the natural process of aging that occurs with the passage of time. *Extrinsic,* or external, aging is intrinsic aging compounded by external factors.

Intrinsic aging is universal and inevitable. As you reach your thirties, your body's production of collagen and elastin, which are important for skin firmness and elasticity, begins to slow down. This is triggered by genetic codes in your DNA and accelerated by changes in hormone levels. The genes you've inherited control intrinsic aging. Some people have genes that allow them to look young far longer than others do. Their hair keeps its color and their skin stays firm and smooth. Generally, a healthy lifestyle is all that is needed for people with good aging genes to remain young looking.

Unfortunately, external or extrinsic factors can accelerate the process of aging, making you look years older than you are—or years older than you would look if your intrinsic aging process had occurred without extrinsic influence. Eight external factors are generally blamed for causing premature aging: sun exposure, cigarette smoking, poor nutrition, air pollution, food allergies, infection, contact allergies, and contact with irritants or toxins. Of these eight, only two are consistently related to premature aging of the skin: sun exposure and cigarette smoking. Doctors at the AAD (2000b) identify overexposure to the sun as a leading cause of age-related skin problems.

Understanding Your Skin

Skin is the largest organ of the human body. It serves numerous functions, including maintaining body temperature and acting as a barrier to harmful elements in your environment. Skin blocks chemicals, toxins, and pollutants and inhibits bacteria from growing. It protects internal organs against contamination and injury. It also produces and stores vitamin D, which is essential for the absorption of calcium and phosphorous, which maintain healthy bone tissue. Finally, the skin has a network of nerves running through it, allowing you to touch and feel sensations such as pain, heat, and cold.

Skin is composed of three layers: the epidermis, the dermis, and the subcutaneous layer.

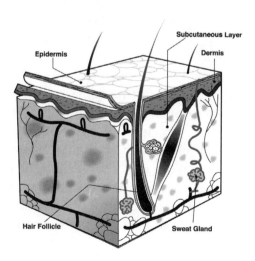

figure 3.1: Cross Section of the Skin

Photosensitivity is an uncommon reaction of the skin or eyes to UVR.

The Epidermis

The *epidermis* is the outer layer or the top layer of skin and is made up of overlapping cells, which create a protective barrier. When the epidermis is healthy, it renews itself every twenty-eight days by shedding older cells and replacing them with newer cells that move up from a lower level within the epidermis called the *basal cell layer*.

Basal cells divide and become *squamous cells*, which are progressively flatter and harder as they move upward toward the surface of the skin. Eventually they rest on the surface, only to be shed and replaced again during the twenty-eight-day cycle.

The *melanocyte* is another important cell contained in the epidermis. This is the cell that produces and distributes *melanin*, the substance also known as *pigment* that gives skin and hair its color. Melanin is the skin's most important defense against the damaging effects of UVR. Amounts of melanin range from minimal in fair skin to very dense in black skin. The abundant melanin in darker skin absorbs much of the UVR energy, helping to prevent damage. (Please be aware, however, that this does not mean people of color do not get skin cancer. We'll discuss this more in chapters 5 and 6.) Skin with low melanin content—fair skin typical of people with blond or red hair and blue or green eyes—is more susceptible to sun damage.

Langerhans cells, found within the epidermis, appear to play an important role in the body's immune system. They protect against tumors, viruses, and other infections and may help prevent skin cancer (Kenet and Lawler 1998).

When UVR strikes the epidermis, it interrupts the cycle that keeps this layer of skin healthy. Some scientists believe that when UVR damages Langerhans cells, a breakdown occurs in the immune system, which then allows for the formation of skin cancers. Others believe that it is the mutations and proliferation of melanocytes resulting from UVR exposure that causes skin cancer in the epidermis. Regardless of which theory is correct, experts agree that chronic UVR exposure causes severe damage to the epidermis, which can result in premature aging, basal cell carcinomas, squamous cell carcinomas, and melanoma.

Photosensitivity can cause an exaggerated
sunburnlike condition (Reid 1996).

The Dermis

Just below the epidermis is the *dermis,* or the second layer of skin. This layer contains blood vessels, lymph vessels, and nerves but is mostly made up of bundles of protein called *collagen.* Collagen keeps skin filled out or wrinkle free by providing support. As you age, you naturally lose some collagen, but exposure to UVR accelerates this process, giving the skin a thin appearance. *Elastin* is also found in the dermis, and, as the name suggests, it gives the skin its elastic qualities. When healthy, the fibers that make up elastin can be stretched 100 percent or more and still return to their original size (Kenet and Lawler 1998). Exposure to UVR breaks down elastin, causing the skin to sag and form wrinkles.

The combined loss of collagen and elastin will gradually make the skin look like old leather. Furthermore, UVR damage to the dermis causes blood vessel swelling *(telangiectases)* and inflammatory white cell accumulation.

The Subcutaneous Layer

The *subcutaneous layer* of the skin is the deepest layer and contains mostly fat. It varies in thickness from person to person and at different parts of the body. This layer of skin acts as insulation, protecting the internal organs from injury while maintaining body temperature.

. . . .

Photoaging and Photodamage

Many people still do not know that they are able to slow down the process of aging just by protecting themselves from the sun. Yet photoaging or photodamage is a condition that doctors have long

Photosensitivity can increase your chances of
getting skin cancer (Reid 1996).

regarded as serious. Not only do people look older with increased lines and wrinkles, but also photoaged skin is a red flag for later development of skin cancers.

Photoaging and photodamage are used interchangeably to describe the chronic changes in the appearance and function of the skin caused by repeated sun exposure rather than by the passage of time. Photoaging occurs when UVR from the sun strikes the skin, creating sunburns and tans at the epidermal level by triggering reactions in the melanocytes, basal cells, and squamous cells and killing some of these cells. UVA particularly has been shown to create damage not only to the epidermis but also to the dermis. This damage could include a breakdown of collagen and elastin and could trigger a cascade of by-products capable of further damage to surrounding tissue. The result is premature aging or photoaging, skin precancers, and cancers.

Skin Conditions Associated with Photoaging

The following skin conditions are specifically associated with damage to the skin caused by UVR.

Wrinkles. As skin ages, the two substances that give it firmness are diminished. Collagen breaks down and elastin weakens. Simultaneously, gravity pulls and the skin sags, making wrinkles. Chronic exposure to the sun or other sources of UVR accelerates this process. Therefore, the more UVR you have been exposed to over your lifetime, the more wrinkled you will look.

Age spots. Age spots are also called "liver spots." They have nothing to do with the liver but rather are associated with chronic sun exposure and age. Flat and brown in appearance, age spots are usually found on the face, hands, back, and feet—areas that are most often exposed to UVR.

Some of the most common age spots are red or brown scaly areas called *actinic keratoses*. Actinic keratoses, which are often called

Some plants, fruits, and medications are photosensitizers.

a precancer, can be easily treated, but if they are ignored, they may eventually become squamous cell skin cancers that need to be removed surgically before they spread throughout the body.

Broken capillaries. "Broken capillaries" or *telangiectasia* are easily seen and appear as a blotchy or ruddy complexion. While everyone experiences dilated facial blood vessels to some degree at some time, chronic sun exposure exacerbates the condition.

Basal cell carcinoma. *Basal cell carcinoma* is a skin cancer that develops at the lowest layer of the epidermis. It often appears as no more than a tiny pinprick or shiny bump on the top of the head, the nose, the face, the neck, or the chest that bleeds and crusts over. Basal cell carcinoma seldom spreads to other parts of the body but can be disfiguring if not treated early. Again, like the other skin conditions associated with photoaging, basal cell carcinoma appears to be directly related to exposure to UVR. (We'll discuss basal cell carcinoma in more detail in chapter 5.)

Squamous cell carcinoma. *Squamous cell carcinoma* is a skin cancer that develops in the uppermost layers of the epidermis and, over time, in the squamous cell layer. It usually appears on the areas of the body that have been most often exposed to the sun: the face, the backs of the hands, the rims of the ears, or the lips. (Older outdoor workers have high rates of squamous cell carcinoma.) This cancer is easy to treat and remove in its early stages. However, if it is ignored, it is capable of spreading to other organs and can eventually be fatal. (We'll discuss squamous cell carcinoma in more detail in chapter 5.)

Melanoma. Melanoma is the deadliest skin cancer. It is associated with aging and sun exposure, although it can develop at any time on anyone. It forms in the epidermis and dermis, and if it is not removed in its early stages, it will spread throughout the body. (We'll discuss melanoma in chapter 6.)

Welding arcs can exceed UVR exposure limits in seconds.

Preventing Photoaging

People who are repeatedly exposed to UVR are at a high risk of photoaging and the skin conditions associated with it. They include people who:

* burn easily, especially those with fair to olive skin and light to medium hair and eyes;

* are outdoors for long periods, either for work or for leisure;

* use tanning beds or sunlamps;

* use medications that cause sun sensitivity; or

* undergo radiation treatment for skin problems.

The best way to prevent photoaging and skin cancers is to protect yourself and your children from UVR by avoiding unprotected sun exposure, especially between 10:00 A.M. and 4:00 P.M.; wearing sun protective clothing and seeking shade; and using broad-spectrum sunscreen with an SPF of 30 or higher, reapplying it every two hours. Even if you already have sun-damaged skin, you will benefit from sun protection.

Treatments for Photoaging

People around the world have used plants, oils, creams, lotions, plastic surgery, and even acupuncture in an effort to prevent and reverse signs of aging. Unfortunately, regardless of which treatment you use, much of the damage caused by the sun is permanent. Some treatments will minimize the symptoms, such as lines, wrinkles, and discoloration, and often can have wonderful results. However, no treatment will work without sun protection. Prevention really is the best treatment.

Tanning lamps generally must exceed occupational limits for UVR exposure in order to cause tanning.

The U.S. Cosmetics Industry: A Brief History

In 2002 the American cosmetics and beauty aid industry totaled over $20 billion in annual sales. Close to $400 million of that was spent on antiaging creams and lotions, all promising softer, younger-looking skin. Demand for all the different types of antiaging products is projected to rise to $25 billion by 2007 (MarketResearch.com 2002).

It took many years for the cosmetics industry to grow to its current size. In the nineteenth century, cleanliness and moral living were encouraged as the best ways to improve appearance, and most women knew how to make simple skin and hair preparations from natural ingredients on their own. Commercial beauty aids were not common, so women drew upon their own therapeutic traditions, using herbs, berries, and other natural substances to care for their skin.

It was not until the later part of the nineteenth century that cosmetics were commercialized. By then chemists, perfumeries, beauty salons, drugstores, mail-order houses, and department stores all recognized the value of beauty products. Elizabeth Arden and Helena Rubinstein, both immigrants from relatively poor families, understood the importance of beauty to a rising middle class, and in a clever marketing move, they provided skin treatments—moisturizing spas, ointments, lotions, and makeup. Their names became synonymous with beauty products to make women look younger. Today these products are still sold, and beauty continues to be measured by how young you look. The younger you look, the more successful or wealthy you appear.

Tanning became a fashion statement before people were aware of the harmful consequences. Most of us now live with symptoms of photoaging, and the pharmaceutical and cosmetics industries are earning billions of dollars helping us try to reverse our mistakes. Perhaps by the time the last baby boomer turns sixty, we will know enough to protect ourselves when we are in the sun and to teach our children to be AWARE. Our grandchildren could have younger-looking, smoother skin well into old age.

Most lamps used for lighting are made to emit little or no UVR.

. . . .

How to Protect Your Skin and Help Reverse Signs of Damage

Be AWARE that you can protect your skin from UVR and immediately help repair damaged skin cells. The effects of any treatment or procedure will last only if skin is protected against UVR.

Sunscreens

Sunscreens are vitally important to preventing and reversing symptoms of photoaging or sun damage. Many dermatologists now recommend that you apply sunscreen every morning before going out and reapply it throughout the day. Sunscreen, particularly broad-spectrum sunscreen that protects the skin from both UVA and UVB with an SPF of 30 or higher, helps protect sun-damaged skin from further exposure and is considered one of the most effective rejuvenators on the market. The less you expose your skin to the sun, the easier it is for cells to repair themselves.

It is important to understand as much as possible about how sunscreens work and why there is growing controversy about how they are used. We have devoted chapter 11 to this topic.

Treatments

There are thousands of prescriptions, procedures, creams, lotions, vitamins, and other assorted remedies that help repair sun-damaged skin. The best advice is to talk to your doctor, dermatologist, or other specialist, who will help you understand your skin type and condition and will inform you about any possible risks before recommending a treatment.

In general, the types of treatments available include retinoids, vitamin C, vitamin E, alpha hydroxy acids, glycolic acids, chemical peels, dermabrasion, microdermabrasion, laser treatments, Botox (botulinum toxin), collagen creams and injections, and plastic surgery.

Sunstroke is caused by dehydration and overheating.

Results of specific treatments will vary according to the condition of an individual's skin. Using creams and lotions—regardless of ingredients—to reduce fine lines, wrinkles, dark circles, age spots, or other symptoms of photoaging will generally take four to eight weeks. If you have allowed this much time and see no results, you should probably try something different.

Faster results require professional procedures. Chemical peels, dermabrasion, and laser peels can be very effective. These procedures may require both preliminary and follow-up treatments to achieve the best results. You should be sure to find out exactly what these treatments are, how long the recovery period will last, how long the results will last, and what possible side effects there are. A consultation with your physician before any procedure will educate you and help determine if a procedure is best for you.

There is no cure for sun-damaged skin, and there are no treatments that can completely reverse the damage. However, many of these products and procedures do help reduce the symptoms or slow down the onset of symptoms. No treatment will be effective without continued sun protection.

Summing Up

Exposure to UVR, whether from the sun or artificial, accelerates the process of aging, making your skin look years older. Sun protection can help prevent, slow down, and even reverse these symptoms of photoaging. The advice of dermatologists and specialists around the world is to use effective sun protection every day and to combine any treatment you may choose to reverse signs of photoaging with ongoing sun protection.

Outdoor workers experience twice the number of nonmelanoma cancers as indoor workers (Conlan 2003).

statistics describe an epidemic of sun damage

Statistics are a fast way to see why skin cancer is considered a growing epidemic and why the numbers of diagnosed melanomas are particularly alarming. Statistics help illustrate the importance of sun protection.

Where Cancer Statistics Come From

The primary authority on cancer statistics in the United States is the National Cancer Institute (NCI). NCI manages a program called Surveillance, Epidemiology, and End Results (SEER) that gives data on cancer incidence, mortality, and patient survival for more than twenty different cancers and for all cancers combined. Using this information, institutions and individuals around the country are able to identify and focus on particular cancer problems, compare and contrast different cancers, identify trends, and draw conclusions. The SEER report is a valuable tool for all cancer research. We have used it to look at the numbers of skin cancers diagnosed, particularly melanoma, and to compare those numbers to other cancers.

While NCI and other similar organizations gather information on melanoma, breast cancer, prostate cancer, lung cancer, and certain other cancers, they do not gather information about basal cell carcinoma or squamous cell carcinoma. The statistics we have for these disorders in the United States are based on smaller samples and therefore are somewhat less reliable than for melanoma.

We have used several other important databases to put together the statistics about skin cancer. These include data from individual hospitals, The Skin Cancer Foundation, the American Association for Cancer Research, the AAD, and the American Cancer Society. While we have not always used this data directly, we value its importance in the research of skin cancer and in providing information for this book.

We have used our own questionnaires and surveys to obtain statistical information from dermatologists about sun protection and patient behaviors. We have also used data from Australia, including data from the Australian Institute of Health and Welfare, the Australasian Association of Cancer Registries, the Australian Radiation Protection and Nuclear Safety Agency, SunSmart Australia, and the National Non-Melanoma Skin Cancer Surveys.

. . . .

An Overview of Skin Cancer in the United States

When you look at the three main types of skin cancer—basal cell carcinoma, squamous cell carcinoma, and melanoma—as a group, some interesting facts emerge. Figure 4.1 shows the number of cases diagnosed for each type of skin cancer in the United States. Figure 4.2 shows the number of deaths from each type of cancer.

Outdoor workers often do not recognize the need to protect themselves.

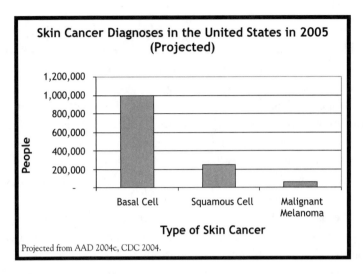

figure 4.1: Skin Cancer Diagnoses in the United States in 2005 (Projected)

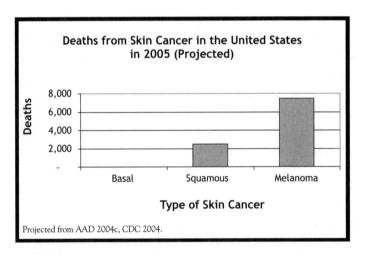

figure 4.2: Deaths from Skin Cancer in the United States in 2005 (Projected)

Basal Cell Carcinoma

Basal cell carcinoma is by far the most common form of skin cancer, accounting for an estimated 1 million of the 1.3 million plus skin cancer diagnoses each year (CDC 2004). This form of skin

Outdoor work can be scheduled to avoid
direct sunlight during peak UV hours.

cancer is easily diagnosed and treated, and while it can be disfiguring, it is primarily considered a cosmetic problem. In fact, most scientific reports about cancer in America do not include basal cell carcinoma.

Squamous Cell Carcinoma

Squamous cell carcinoma accounts for about 16 percent of diagnosed cases of skin cancer each year. It is also considered primarily a cosmetic problem, but if left untreated it becomes deadly. Approximately 2,340 Americans die of squamous cell carcinoma and other nonmelanoma skin cancers each year (AAD 2004c).

Melanoma

Melanoma has the smallest number of diagnosed cases each year. However, it is the most deadly. The survival rate for melanoma is similar to that for breast cancer or prostate cancer—it eventually kills between one in four and one in five people diagnosed with *malignant* (invasive) melanoma. More than 55,000 Americans were diagnosed with malignant melanoma in 2004. Approximately 40,780 were diagnosed *in situ* (noninvasive). Approximately 7,910 will die from the disease—5,050 men and 2,860 women (AAD 2004b).

The single most important statistic about melanoma is its growth rate: approximately 4 to 5 percent per year since 2003 (AAD 2004b). Figure 4.3 shows per capita melanoma rates for men and women from 1973 to 1998. If melanoma were like lung cancer or colon cancer, the lines would actually be sloping down. If melanoma were just growing at the same rate as the U.S. population, then the lines in the chart would be flat. But the lines for melanoma are aggressively rising. These statistics show that the numbers of diagnosed cases of melanoma are growing at an epidemic rate.

Who Is Affected by Melanoma?

Statistics from NCI's SEER Public Use Data (2001) provide a clear profile of the people affected by melanoma in America today.

Outdoor work can be shared to cut down individual exposure time.

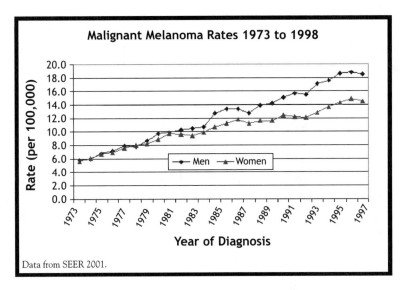

figure 4.3: Malignant Melanoma Rates 1973 to 1993

White-skinned people are affected by melanoma more often than dark-skinned people. Your skin color and type says a lot about your susceptibility to melanoma. People with darker skin have more melanin and are naturally better protected against the UVR that causes melanoma. According to the AAD (2004b), Caucasians are ten times more likely than people of other races to be diagnosed with melanoma, while the American Cancer Society (2004b) calculates that melanoma risk is twenty times higher for Caucasians than for African-Americans. The lack of melanin in white skin makes it more susceptible to the damage caused by the sun.

However, while African-Americans still have a lower incidence of diagnosed melanoma, studies have shown that their long-term survival is significantly lower than that of Caucasians, 58.8 percent as compared to 84.8 percent (Taylor and Rahman 2001). This is attributed to the disease being detected at later and more dangerous stages.

Middle-aged to elderly people are affected by melanoma more often than young people. Melanoma is most commonly diagnosed in people in their forties though seventies—baby boomers and seniors. This is the result of intense and cumulative exposure to the sun's

Make use of shaded work areas when possible.

UVR. In other words, a lifetime of sun exposure, particularly a lot of exposure when you are young, adds up and eventually overcomes your skin's ability to repair itself. This loss of recuperative powers most typically leads to melanoma in the forty-to-seventy-nine age range. Figure 4.4 shows malignant melanoma diagnoses by age group.

A part of the reason that melanoma will continue to grow aggressively in the coming decades is the aging baby boom generation. Within two decades, the number of people over fifty in America is predicted to be 36 percent or more of the total population (Population Reference Bureau 2000).

Men are affected by melanoma more often than women. Typically, three men are diagnosed with melanoma for every two women (Beddingfield et al. 2002). This is partly because more men work outdoors. In addition, women do a much better job protecting themselves from the sun. As a group, men avoid using sun protection products such as sunscreen.

Among people with the same skin type, those living closer to the equator are affected by melanoma more often than those living at higher latitudes. There is a basic relationship between

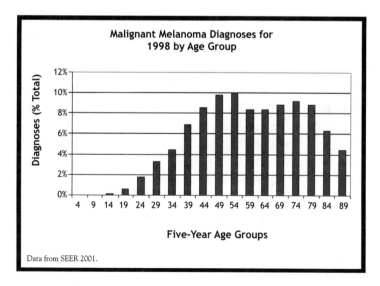

figure 4.4: Malignant Melanoma Diagnoses for 1998 by Age Group

Shade structures for work and play will help prevent skin cancer.

latitude and skin cancer rates. However, while it would seem an easy prediction to say that the Sun Belt states should lead the United States in per capita melanoma rates, they don't. The states with the highest per capita melanoma rates are, in descending order, Connecticut, Oregon, Colorado, Utah, Washington state, and Idaho (SEER 2001).

The most important contributing factor to the number of melanoma cases in these states is skin type. There is a higher percentage of white people in these states than in the Sun Belt states, illustrating that as a risk factor, skin type outweighs the effect of the greater UVR exposure in the Sun Belt. However, when comparing the number of cases within only the white population of all states, the highest melanoma rates are in Hawaii and California, as you would expect based on their geographic location (SEER 2001).

The Cost of Treating Melanoma and Other Skin Cancers

A study by Tsao, Rogers, and Sober (1998) estimated that the annual direct cost of treating melanoma in the United States was $563 million. The study also found that 90 percent of this total annual cost could be attributed to less than 20 percent of patients: those patients with advanced disease, that is, stage III and stage IV melanoma that required extensive treatment. Stage I and stage II patients each represented just 5 percent of the total cost.

Bringing this analysis forward to 2005, by adjusting for the greater number of melanoma patients and an approximate 10 percent annual rise in the cost of medicine, the direct cost of treating newly diagnosed melanoma would be $1.5 billion for 2005. In addition, in Australia, Mathers and colleagues (1998) estimated that the direct costs of treating nonmelanoma skin cancers were five times the costs associated with treating melanoma. Assuming the ratio of melanoma cases to nonmelanoma cases in Australia is similar to the ratio in the United States, then the direct cost of treating sun-related skin cancer in America is approximately $9 billion per year.

This figure is conservative. It does not take into account the cost of screening, education, lost time at work, patient home care,

Employee awareness of skin cancer is important for prevention.

and patient investment in plastic surgery or skincare products. Nor does it reflect rises in insurance premiums or settlements paid by employers. It does not reflect the loss of income due to death. We estimate that adding these indirect costs would increase the total to significantly more than $10 billion for 2005. Skin cancer is having a huge and still growing economic impact in the United States.

· ·
Melanoma in the Future

The numbers of diagnosed cases of some major forms of cancer, such as lung cancer and colon cancer, have stabilized or are actually declining. Melanoma, in contrast, is on an exponential growth track. If the current trends continue unchanged over the next decade, melanoma will become more common in the white population, especially in the Sun Belt, than lung cancer or colon cancer.

Lessons from Australia

In 1988 state governments in Australia began to aggressively support public education about sun protection, funding these programs at levels significantly higher than current spending on similar programs in the United States. Unfortunately, it took ten years before the earliest evidence of any decrease in melanoma rates could be seen in people under fifty in Australia. There was no decline in melanoma rates for people over fifty, although there were declines in the death rate (Carter, Marks, and Hill 1999). This demonstrated that public education aimed at preventing melanoma is a process that takes several decades—a process only just beginning in America.

To our benefit, Australians discovered the relationship between sun exposure in childhood and later skin cancers. (We'll discuss sun exposure in children in chapter 8.) This awareness led to an unprecedented education and prevention campaign targeting children, parents, and teachers as well as physicians and other health-care workers, local governments, and trade unions. The campaign was

Even when it is cool and cloudy, outdoor workers are at risk from UVR.

heavily supported by the media, which provided consistent and constant reminders about the importance of using sun protection.

Nearly two decades later, Australia is able to demonstrate positive statistical changes in melanoma rates. There are now fewer melanoma cases being diagnosed in people younger than fifty, and melanomas are being detected and treated at earlier stages in older people (AIHW and AACR 2000).

Sun Protection Education in the United States

Within the United States, the states that will be most affected by the melanoma epidemic will be those with high percentages of white-skinned residents, those with high percentages of seniors, and those located within the Sun Belt. In addition to the strain on state health programs, the already struggling national health-care system, Medicare/Medicaid, will need to accommodate an epidemic of melanoma among seniors.

From a public health perspective, the solution to this rising epidemic of melanoma is commitment to a well-funded, long-term primary prevention campaign. The Australian experience with programs like SunSmart has shown that public education will eventually lead to a decline in melanoma rates in those under fifty but that it takes decades for this type of change. Additional public education programs should be developed to help those over fifty identify and seek treatment for melanoma earlier, leading to a decline in the death rate from melanoma. Further, since we now know that unprotected exposure at any time can trigger the biological reaction leading to skin cancer, education campaigns should be targeted to all age groups.

If the United States increases public education spending on sun protection from its current modest level to match the recommended per capita spending within Australia, it would involve a commitment of $75 million annually across the country for the next fifteen to twenty years. This investment could be fully funded by a tax of 2 percent on the use of tanning beds, which would provide $100 million

On the equinox (about March 21 and September 23), day and night are of equal length.

annually. A study by Carter, Marks, and Hill (1999) suggests that as the rate of melanoma declines, this spending on public education could show a return of three dollars in benefits for every dollar invested.

How many years will it take for America to decide to significantly increase spending on public health education about sun protection? Again, if we look at what happened in Australia, some state governments will aggressively fund public health education, while many others will lag behind. Perhaps, like antismoking programs, state campaigns should be combined with federal legislative action.

Summing Up

The number of diagnosed skin cancers, particularly melanoma, has been rising dramatically in America over the past twenty-five years. Statistics show the increases and the consequences. Education about prevention and detection is the only way to lower the numbers and slow the epidemic.

The winter solstice (around December 22) is the shortest day of the year.

* 5 *

nonmelanoma skin cancers

Unlike melanoma, nonmelanoma skin cancers are generally not fatal. While primarily a cosmetic problem, they should not be taken lightly. Over a million Americans developed nonmelanoma skin cancers in 2004, and 2,340 died from the disease (AAD 2004c). If detected early, nonmelanoma skin cancer can almost always be treated, removed, and cured.

. . . .

Causes of Nonmelanoma Skin Cancers

The AAD, The Skin Cancer Foundation, and other cancer organizations around the world agree that actinic keratoses, a precancerous skin condition, and the two most common nonmelanoma skin cancers—basal cell carcinoma and squamous cell carcinoma—are primarily caused by unprotected exposure to UVR. Further, the most significant predisposing factor for all three of these conditions is fair skin. People who have fair to olive skin and light to medium hair and eyes are at highest risk. People of color also get these skin cancers, particularly squamous cell carcinoma, which is known to develop on the surface of old scars and skin injuries.

There are other factors that contribute to these skin cancers: exposure to artificial UVR from tanning beds; heredity; prolonged suppression of the immune system; exposure to X-rays; prolonged contact with coal, tar, pitch, or arsenic compounds; and complications from burns, scars, vaccinations, and even tattoos. However, the overriding factor that both causes and compounds these diseases is exposure to the harmful rays of the sun.

The Three Major Types of Nonmelanoma Skin Cancer

In this chapter, we'll take a look at the symptoms, diagnosis, and treatment of the three major kinds of nonmelanoma skin cancer: actinic keratoses, basal cell carcinoma, and squamous cell carcinoma.

Actinic Keratoses

Actinic keratoses are most often associated with older, fair-skinned people who have been chronically exposed to the sun. They generally appear on skin that is least often covered by clothing—the hands, face, tips of ears, scalp, and forearms. Actinic keratoses affect at least 10 million Americans, and they are especially prevalent among people who live in sunny climates (AAD 2003). Most dermatologists think of this disease as a precancerous skin condition. Actinic keratoses are an alteration of epidermal cells called *keratinocytes*, and while they take years to develop, they ultimately become highly visible. Given that "cancer" is a general term used to describe diseases characterized by abnormal changes in cells, actinic keratoses are usually included in descriptions of nonmelanoma skin cancers.

The summer solstice (around June 21) is the longest day of the year.

Symptoms

Actinic keratoses are small bumps with rough, scaly surfaces or sores. They can be as little as the tip of a pencil or as large as a quarter. A person can have one or several at the same time. Some older patients find that they must be treated periodically for these lesions over many years. If this happens, your physician will carefully monitor the lesions and may give different treatments accordingly.

Diagnosis

Diagnosis is usually easy because the lesions have unique physical characteristics that physicians can identify by visual examination. Occasionally, if the lesion is especially large or thick, it will need to be surgically removed for microscopic examination (*biopsy*) to determine if it has changed to cancer. If cancerous, actinic keratoses will likely be diagnosed as squamous cell carcinoma.

Treatment

Once the diagnosis is made, dermatologists will consider a number of factors before choosing the most appropriate methods of treatment. Some of these factors include

* the location, size, and number of lesions;

* the desired cosmetic outcome;

* the patient's age, health, and medical history;

* the patient's ability to comply with treatment; and

* the patient's history of previous treatments.

If diagnosed in the early stages, actinic keratoses can be removed by *cryotherapy* (freezing), surgical excision, or *curettage* (scraping); by applying a cream (Aldara, or imiquimod); or by chemical peeling, dermabrasion, laser surgery, or other dermatologic

While less intense than direct UVR, indirect UVR can still damage skin.

surgical procedures. (We'll describe many of these procedures in more detail later in this chapter and in chapter 6.)

Actinic keratoses can be prevented by using sun protection early and throughout life. Since it is cited as one of the most common reasons to consult a dermatologist (AAD 2003), it is probably one of the more notable drains on Medicare and other insurance. Education about prevention and detection should eventually lower the number of people with this disease.

As we mentioned, actinic keratosis is a precancer that can turn into cancer if left untreated. Having it treated and removed is vitally important to the prevention of cancer. If you develop any of the symptoms described above, see your dermatologist.

Basal Cell Carcinoma

More Americans develop basal cell carcinoma (BCC) than any other skin cancer. In 2004 there were 800,000 Americans affected by this cancer, and while the majority of those affected are older men, women are getting BCC more frequently than in the past (SCF 2004a).

Basal cell carcinoma forms in the basal cells of the epidermis. As you'll remember from chapter 3, the basal cell layer is where the new cells of the epidermis are formed, then pushed to the surface to replace old cells during a twenty-eight-day cycle.

When the layer of basal cells is repeatedly exposed to UVR, a biochemical process is set into action that causes mutations, overproduction of cells, and eventually basal cell carcinoma. These damaged or cancerous cells are still pushed to the surface but present themselves as lesions and tumors. The tumors have common characteristics that are easily recognized.

Symptoms

There are five warning signs of basal cell carcinoma that you can easily look for when you examine your skin:

* a sore that does not heal

Sunburn from reflected or scattered UVR can occur in shaded areas.

* a persistent irritated or reddish patch that may be sensitive and itch

* a translucent bump or nodule that is sometimes confused with a mole but is usually pink, white, or pearly in color

* a small growth, usually pink, with a crusted center surrounded by a slightly elevated, rolled border

* a white, yellow, or waxy area that looks scarlike with poorly defined borders

Diagnosis

If you have recognized any of the warning signs for BCC, it is important that you immediately contact your primary care physician or dermatologist. Your doctor will examine the growth and evaluate your medical history, then decide whether or not to perform a biopsy. In most states, physicians are liable for missed diagnosis, so you can expect that your doctor will recommend a biopsy if anything looks suspicious. Be sure to tell your doctor if any other member of your family has had skin cancer or if you are taking any medications that can make you sun sensitive. Sometimes a second biopsy is needed to confirm a diagnosis. Don't be alarmed by this. It is always better to be safe than sorry.

A biopsy is usually a fast and painless procedure performed by your doctor in the office. After injecting a local anesthetic and waiting for the area to become numb, your doctor will remove all of or a sample of the growth so that it can be examined under a microscope and treatment can be determined.

Since basal cell carcinoma rarely *metastasizes*, or spreads to other organs, formal staging is not usually necessary. Your dermatologist will likely recommend a procedure he or she feels will effectively rid your skin of the cancer while causing the least amount of cosmetic harm.

Basal cell carcinoma can recur in the same place, or new basal cell cancers can start in other locations. As many as 40 percent of patients diagnosed with one basal cell carcinoma will develop a new

Snow and sand have high UVR reflection levels.

skin cancer within a few years of the first diagnosis (AAD 2000a). It is extremely important, therefore, to continue to routinely check your whole body for suspicious lesions. Basal cell carcinoma rarely spreads to other organs but can cause local destruction or disfiguration if not treated in time.

Treatment

There are several standard methods for removing BCC. Which method you use should be decided with your doctor and will depend on whether the tumor is *primary* (first time) or *recurrent* as well as on its location, size, and type. The outcome of any treatment relies heavily on these factors as well as on the surgeon's skills.

The first three procedures listed below are reasonably easy, have cure rates as high as 95 percent, and have good cosmetic outcomes (that is, minimal scarring). However, these procedures are only effective for treating primary BCC.

Aldara. Known generically as imiquimod, Aldara is an immune response modifier. It comes in a cream form and is applied five days a week for six weeks. Aldara has only recently been approved by the Food and Drug Administration to treat superficial BCC on the body, neck, arms, or legs, but not on the face. The cure rate is about 80 percent (FDA 2004). Using Aldara in combination with other treatments may push up the success rate for the cream.

Electrodesiccation and curettage. This procedure is short and simple. Your doctor will numb the area with anesthesia, then carefully scrape the tumor out using a scooplike instrument called a *curette*. After the tumor is removed, the surrounding base and margins are cauterized with a heat-producing electric needle. This is a highly effective treatment for primary and superficial BCC. Cure rates are as high as 95 percent.

Cryosurgery. This is an option only for those who have superficial BCC. Cryosurgery has good cosmetic outcomes (little scarring) and good cure rates. Liquid nitrogen is applied to the tumor, which then freezes, destroying the cancerous cells.

Snow can reflect as much as 80 percent of UVR that hits it (NZDS 2004).

The following procedures are used for more advanced or more serious basal cell carcinomas. Cure rates are as high as 95 percent.

Surgical excision. This procedure is often short and simple. Unfortunately, healing times are longer, and the cosmetic outcome may be poor. After a local anesthetic has taken effect, a scalpel is used to make an incision down to the subcutaneous level of the skin, increasing the likelihood that the complete tumor will be removed. Surrounding layers of the epidermis and dermis are also likely to be removed. This leaves a larger scar but increases the cure rate.

Mohs micrographically controlled surgery. This is a time-consuming surgery, but it has the highest cure rate and it spares as much uninvolved skin as possible. After anesthesia is given, the surgeon removes thin layers of the tumor, one at a time, checking each under a microscope for malignant cells. The procedure stops when a layer that is free of cancer cells is reached. Controlled removal of tissue minimizes scarring and is often used for recurrent lesions or BCC in difficult places (around the nose or near the eyes).

Ionizing radiation or radiation therapy. This procedure is usually reserved for older patients, who may not tolerate extensive or difficult surgical procedures. It is good for facial tumors, although less effective for nonfacial tumors. Superficial radiation is directed at the malignant cells, requiring as many as ten treatments to destroy the tumor.

Scarring

Patients usually wonder whether the scars resulting from surgery can be "fixed." The answer is generally yes, to a certain extent. After a skin cancer has been removed from a cosmetically important part of the body, such as the face, reconstructive surgery using a skin flap or skin graft may be performed. If you are concerned about scarring, you should consult a plastic surgeon.

Sea surf can reflect as much as 25 percent of UVR (NZDS 2004).

Squamous Cell Carcinoma

More than 250,000 diagnoses of squamous cell carcinoma are made in the United States each year, making it the second most common form of skin cancer (AAD 2000c). Like BCC, squamous cell carcinoma starts in the epidermis, but in the keratinocytes rather than in the basal cells. These cells are at the top layer of the epidermis and become highly visible when altered or malignant. Squamous cell carcinoma can develop from actinic keratoses, and while this cancer usually spreads only within the epidermis and upper dermis, it can eventually penetrate the lower levels of the skin and, if not treated, will metastasize to distant tissues and organs. Approximately 2,500 deaths in United States are attributed to squamous cell carcinoma each year (AAD 2000c). However, the more common effect of leaving these cancers untreated is serious disfigurement. The spreading malignancy will destroy much of the tissue surrounding the original tumor, which can result in the loss of the nose or an ear.

Symptoms

Generally, squamous cell carcinomas—like basal cell carcinomas and actinic keratoses—are found on areas of the body that have been repeatedly exposed to UVR: the scalp, backs of hands, rims of ears, lips, shoulders, arms, and back. They can also be found, however, anywhere on the body, including inside the mouth and on the genitalia.

Symptoms for squamous cell carcinoma include patches of skin that are wartlike, crusted, or inflamed and sometimes bleed; sores that don't heal; or growths that have central indentations and bleed or increase in size. If you have any of these symptoms, or if you are concerned about a lesion that is changing, you should see your primary care physician or dermatologist.

Diagnosis

Squamous cell carcinomas usually enlarge slowly, but they can easily invade neighboring tissue. The only way to determine whether

Shade is at a maximum in the middle of a structure.

the skin growth is cancerous is to biopsy it. As we suggested earlier, your dermatologist will likely only need to biopsy once, but do not be alarmed if a second biopsy is asked for.

Once the results are confirmed, squamous cell carcinomas are given a stage. This is because they can spread to other organs of the body, and staging helps the doctor determine which treatment is best.

Stage 0. The cancer is still contained in the epidermis. It has not spread to the dermis nor to the deep subcutaneous layer of skin. Squamous cell cancer at this stage is usually easy to remove. Also in this category are lesions we have described as actinic keratoses.

Stage I. The cancerous growth is no larger than two centimeters (about three-quarters of an inch). It has not spread to lymph nodes or other organs but may have penetrated all three layers of skin. It is still easy to remove, although scarring may occur. Cure rates are high.

Stage II. The growth is larger than two centimeters, but it has not spread to lymph nodes or other organs. Scarring may be a problem. Cure rates are still high.

Stage III. The cancer has spread to tissues beneath the skin (such as muscle, bone, or cartilage), to nearby lymph nodes, or both. The cancer has not yet spread to other organs (such as the lungs, liver, or brain). Treatments will vary. Cure rates are lower.

Stage IV. The cancer can be any size. It has spread to other organs, such as the lungs or brain. Treatments will vary. Cure rates are poor.

Treatment

After a biopsy confirms the presence of squamous cell carcinoma, the tumor must be removed. *It is important to remember that the tumor was not removed with the biopsy.*

Dermatologists and other physicians use a variety of different surgical procedures based on the location, size, and microscopic characteristics of the tumor. Most options are relatively minor office-based

Trees planted in clusters provide the most shade cover.

procedures that require only local anesthesia and have been described in detail in the section on basal cell carcinoma treatments.

The major difference in treatment of the two cancers is that the removal of squamous cell carcinoma will always leave a scar. Often, the scar can be hidden in the skin folds, but squamous cell carcinomas are usually much bigger under the skin than they appear on the surface. That is why the hole left after the removal of the cancer is often bigger than the growth that was visible before the procedure.

If you have had a squamous cell cancer removed, you should be closely monitored by your dermatologist. You should see the doctor for a skin exam every three months for the first two years and then every six months for life.

Summing Up

Nonmelanoma skin cancers are the most common cancers in the United States. They are most often found on areas of the body that are exposed to UVR and could be prevented with effective sun protection methods. When detected and treated early, they can be easily removed with a high cure rate. However, they should not be taken lightly. They can be disfiguring, and if left untreated, some can metastasize to become lethal.

For more information about these cancers, see "Online Resources" at the back of the book.

Most communities must rely on local government
for the provision of shade.

melanoma

Malignant cancers (cancers that have the ability to invade and destroy surrounding cells) are some of the most feared and potentially devastating health problems. However, having the facts about cancer is always the best way to prevent it and to fight it.

Melanoma is deadly, and it is being diagnosed in epidemic numbers. According to The Skin Cancer Foundation (2004b), the incidence of melanoma rose more quickly over the last ten years than the incidence of any other cancer. Melanoma still accounts for only 4 percent of all skin cancers detected, yet every hour one person in the United States dies from the disease. In 2004 an estimated 29,900 men and 25,200 women were diagnosed with melanoma. At these rates, one in sixty-five Americans has a lifetime risk of developing invasive melanoma, while one in thirty-seven will develop noninvasive melanoma (AAD 2004c).

Melanomas are also being diagnosed in younger people more than ever before. While melanoma was once thought of as a cancer of older men, 60 percent of deaths due to melanoma occur in patients younger than sixty, and 20 percent occur in patients younger than forty (Masci and Borden 2002). It is still rare in young children, but melanoma has been found in teenagers and has become more common than any other cancer among women between the ages of twenty-five and twenty-nine (AAD 2004c).

All these facts are alarming. However, early detection and treatment can cure melanoma almost 100 percent of the time (SCF 2004b). If you ignore the symptoms or delay a visit to the doctor, you are surrendering to the enemy before you have begun to fight. Pay attention to your skin. Know the warning signs of melanoma and other skin cancers, and get treatment immediately.

The information in this chapter should not be considered medical advice. You should always consult your doctor if you think you may have melanoma.

What Is Melanoma?

Melanoma usually starts in the epidermis, in the melanocytes, and will grow down into the skin to eventually reach the blood and lymph vessels. From there it spreads to all parts of the body. While melanoma most often starts growing on the surface of the skin, it can also develop in the eye, where it is called *intraocular melanoma,* or in other parts of the body where pigment cells are found. While these kinds of melanoma are extremely rare, the four types of melanoma of the skin have become epidemic.

The Four Basic Types of Melanoma

Melanoma of the skin is categorized into four basic types. The first three begin in a localized area at the surface of the skin and are in situ. These become invasive if left untreated but can generally be cured when treated early. The fourth type of melanoma, *nodular melanoma,* is the most aggressive, and because it is invasive from the start, it is the most dangerous.

Superficial spreading melanoma. While this melanoma is the type most often found among younger patients, it accounts for 70 percent of all melanomas diagnosed (SCF 2004b). It is easy to detect and treat early if you are careful to watch for changes in your skin. Superficial spreading melanoma acts as its name suggests—it spreads along the

Australia has the highest incidence of skin cancer of any country in the world.

surface of the skin before spreading more deeply. It usually takes the form of a flat or slightly raised patch with colors that vary from white to black with irregular borders. It may take the form of an older mole that has changed or a new one that has appeared. It can be found anywhere on the body but is common on the legs of women and on the torsos of men. They are also found on the upper backs and shoulders of both men and women, which suggests that it is important to have someone else periodically check these areas for you.

Lentigo maligna. This melanoma is most often found among the elderly, but like superficial spreading melanoma, it can be found in people of all ages. Fortunately, lentigo maligna stays close to the surface of the skin for some time before penetrating more deeply, which means you can detect it early and treat it before it spreads. It is found on parts of the body that are most often exposed to UVR. It is usually an uneven or mottled tan, brown, or dark brown and appears flat or slightly elevated. Lentigo maligna will become an invasive melanoma if left untreated.

Acral lentiginous melanoma. This melanoma is perhaps one of the most sinister because it is often mistaken for a bruise or other minor skin problem. It is the most common melanoma found in African-Americans (SCF 2004b). It usually appears under the nails or on the soles of the feet or palms of the hands, as a black or brown discoloration. It spreads superficially over the skin before penetrating more deeply. Unfortunately, because most education about skin cancer has not traditionally been directed at dark-skinned people, it is often not detected until its later, more life-threatening stages.

Nodular melanoma. Nodular melanoma is mainly found in the elderly and is perhaps the melanoma most people think of when discussing the disease. This is the most aggressive melanoma, and it is usually invasive by the time it is diagnosed. The malignancy appears as a bump, which is often black but can be tan, red, brown, blue, gray, or white. It is most frequently found on the legs, arms, and torso. Nodular melanoma accounts for 10 to 15 percent of melanoma cases (SCF 2004b).

A UV card is a simple, credit card sized device that indicates UVR intensity.

. . . .
Risk Factors for Melanoma

There are several different risk factors that contribute to the development of melanoma. The three most common are dysplastic nevi, genetic factors, and exposure to UVR. We have included others as well to give you a broad understanding of the risk factors for this disease.

Dysplastic Nevi

Dysplastic nevi or *atypical moles* are different from ordinary or common moles. They are usually larger, flat, and have irregular borders and color. They are present in 2 to 5 percent of Caucasian adults, and they are often the sites of malignant melanoma. However, people who have many moles, whether they are dysplastic or common, appear to be at an increased risk of developing melanoma (Masci and Borden 2002). While most people have some moles—usually around thirty—most are without significance. If you have more than fifty moles, you should be aware that you are in a high risk category for developing melanoma (ACS 2003b). Dysplastic nevi put you in an even higher risk category, and you should carefully monitor your skin.

Genetic Factors

Heredity, or genetic factors, can also put you at a higher risk for melanoma. If a close relative—such as a parent, brother or sister, aunt, or uncle—has had melanoma, then your chances for getting the disease are increased. Approximately 10 percent of people who get melanoma have a family history of the disease (ACS 2004b). Ask your parents or other members of your family if anyone has had melanoma, and routinely check your skin if you are genetically related to someone who has had this disease. Further, be sure that all the members of your family are aware of the risk and routinely checked by a physician.

A UV card measures the strength of UV rays in about twenty seconds.

Exposure to UVR

Whether from the sun or from tanning beds, unprotected exposure to UVR is considered a primary risk factor for melanoma. Researchers have tried to pinpoint the types of exposure that are most harmful and have generally concluded that *any* unprotected exposure creates a risk. If you have a history of tanning or spending a lot of time in the sun, you have a high risk of developing this deadly disease. However, some behaviors are now considered more dangerous than others. Following is a description of some of those behaviors.

Intermittent sun exposure. If you are exposed to UVR sporadically, you may be at a higher risk for developing melanoma (Elwood 1992). A good example of a person with intermittent exposure would be an indoor worker who has only weekends or vacations to be outdoors. Another good example would be a person who occasionally uses a tanning bed.

Chronic sun exposure. If you are outdoors often or continually, exposed to UVR (for example, if you work outdoors), you are at a high risk for all skin cancers, including melanoma.

Cumulative sun exposure. This is the amount of sun exposure or exposure to artificial UVR that has accumulated over a lifetime. It reflects the effects of both intermittent and chronic sun exposure. In other words, you may have been an outdoor worker for ten years, during which time you received chronic sun exposure, then spent ten years working in an office and receiving intermittent sun exposure, all of which adds up to cumulative sun exposure. The more cumulative sun exposure you have had, the higher your chances for developing skin cancer.

While scientists are still researching and debating the full nature of the relationship between UVR and melanoma, it is clear that there is strong relationship—and that avoiding exposure or using effective sun protection methods will help prevent melanoma and other skin cancers. Further, intermittent sun exposure appears to be directly

UVR is primarily responsible for the fading of home furnishings.

correlated to melanoma, and those people receiving intermittent exposure seem to be at the highest risk for developing the disease (Elwood 1992).

Skin Color

Skin color can also put you at a higher risk for melanoma. If you have fair skin and light hair, blue or green eyes, and skin that sunburns easily, you are at a higher risk for developing the disease. You can determine your skin type in chapter 7, and if you find that your skin is type I (pale white or freckled, always burns, never tans) or type II (white, always burns, tans minimally), you should be especially careful to periodically check for signs of melanoma.

People with dark skin also develop melanoma, particularly on the palms of the hands, on the soles of the feet, under the nails, and inside the mouth. African-Americans with melanoma are more likely than whites to have advanced disease—usually acral lentiginous melanoma—at the time of diagnosis (Taylor and Rahman 2001).

Weakened Immune System

Weakening of the immune system may also be a contributing factor to developing melanoma. Exposure to UVA weakens the Langerhans cells, which are part of the immune system. The immune system can also be weakened by other diseases or cancers, by drugs given after organ transplants or after surgery, or by HIV (human immunodeficiency virus), with the result being a poor defense against a developing cancer.

Previous Melanomas

If you have had melanoma diagnosed once, you are at a high risk for developing melanoma again.

Fifty percent of the solar heat entering a home comes in through the windows (Hunter Douglas Windows 2004).

Age

Advanced age does not cause melanoma, but we have included it as a risk factor because middle-aged to elderly people are more likely to be diagnosed with the disease. Therefore, if you are in these age groups, you should carefully check for any early signs of the disease. Further, you should understand that UVR exposure does not have to be recent to put you at a high risk for melanoma. As with other skin cancers, the biological process that leads to melanoma could have been triggered when you were a child, or it could have been triggered last month. Melanoma can be triggered at any age with exposure to UVR (Bulliard 2000) but is likely to appear at later ages. Sun protection should be practiced throughout life.

Lack of Awareness

According to a survey released by the Centers for Disease Control (CDC) and the AAD in 1996, many Americans are unaware of the dangers of melanoma. Of those surveyed, 74 percent between the ages of eighteen and twenty-four did not know what melanoma was, and 42 percent between the ages of twenty-five and forty-four had no knowledge of the disease (AAD and CDC 1996). While this survey is somewhat dated, a more recent study found that fewer than one-third of American youths practiced effective sun protection (Geller et al. 2002). We conducted a survey of dermatologists in 2004 and found that low numbers of patients were using sun protection and that few were aware of melanoma. When people don't know that melanoma exists or what causes it, they are at risk of behavior that may lead to this deadly disease.

Recognizing Melanoma

Melanoma is easily detectable and curable in its early stages. We urge you to make a habit of periodically checking your whole body for any signs of melanoma. It is easy to do, and it may save your life. If you

Reggae singer Bob Marley died of complications from melanoma.

have a question or a concern about something on your skin, you should see your doctor.

This mnemonic, the ABCDs of melanoma, was developed to help you evaluate changes in your moles in order to recognize melanoma at its earliest and potentially curable stage (see figure 6.1). It is used by The Skin Cancer Foundation, the AAD, the National Cancer Institute, and many other institutions and individuals concerned with preventing melanoma. The letter *E* for "evolving" has also become part of much of the literature about melanoma, so we have included it here.

A = Asymmetry. Draw an imaginary line down the middle of any mole and ask yourself if the two halves match. Ordinary moles are usually round and symmetrical, while melanomas are often asymmetrical.

B = Border. Ordinary moles are round or oval and have well-defined, smooth, even borders. Melanomas often have irregular, uneven, or notched borders. Also, pigment spreading from the border of the mole into surrounding skin is a warning sign of melanoma.

C = Color. Ordinary moles are usually one even color throughout and are most often brown, tan, or flesh colored. If your mole has several colors—including black, brown, red, white, and blue—or an irregular pattern of colors, it may be melanoma.

D = Diameter. Watch for a change in the size of your moles. Ordinary moles are generally less than six millimeters (a quarter of an inch) in diameter, or about the diameter of a pencil eraser. Melanomas may be as small as an eighth of an inch, but they are more often larger.

E = Evolving. While *E* for "evolving" is not part of the classic mnemonic, it is important to know that ordinary moles usually do not change over time. A mole that changes in size, shape, shades of color, surface, or

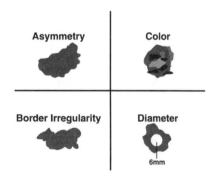

figure 6.1: ABCDs of Melanoma

Actor Burgess Meredith died of complications from melanoma.

symptoms may be suspicious for melanoma. Further, if it tingles, itches, burns, or feels strange, it may be evolving and should be checked.

Other warning signs include a sore that does not heal or any change in the surface of a mole, such as scaliness, oozing, or bleeding. If you have melanoma, you may experience only one of the symptoms described above. You do not need to experience all of these symptoms to have melanoma. Any suspicious change in a mole should be evaluated by a doctor immediately.

. . . .

Full Body Checks

It is important to remember that not everyone who has one or more of the risk factors listed above will get melanoma. It is also important to know that melanoma can develop even if you do not have any of these risk factors. Therefore, you should be AWARE and periodically perform a complete body check to look for symptoms of the disease. Early detection and treatment of melanoma will usually provide a high cure rate. If you know your own skin—its imperfections, freckles, and moles—you will notice changes.

The recommended frequency of self-exams and exams performed by doctors will depend on your risk of getting the disease. Poole and Guerry (1998) recommend monthly self-exams for people with a personal or family history of melanoma or dysplastic nevi, as well as frequent exams (quarterly for people at very high risk) by a dermatologist or other specially trained physician. The Skin Cancer Foundation goes further by recommending that you teach your children to perform self-exams early so they can do it themselves by the time they are teens (SCF 2001).

Men in particular should be encouraged to give themselves body checks, asking someone to help them if needed. The highest number of diagnosed melanomas are found in men, yet men are less likely than women to spot them or seek treatment (Koh et al. 1992).

In Australia there has been a decline in the number of deaths caused by melanoma, and this decline can be directly related to the ongoing campaign over the past twenty years to educate the public

Maureen Reagan, daughter of Ronald Reagan,
died of complications from melanoma.

about prevention, early detection, and treatment. Teaching people how to give themselves a full body check has been part of that campaign.

Articles Needed for a Body Check

To perform this easy task, you will need the following:

* a well-lighted room

* two chairs

* two mirrors, one full-length and one handheld

* blow-dryer

* comb

* notebook

* pencil

You should keep a notebook to keep track of numbers of moles, sizes, and locations. If possible, take photographs, particularly if you have more than fifty moles or if you have dysplastic nevi. This will allow you to document any changes and will make it easier to describe them to your physician. Keep copies of the ABCDs of Melanoma (figure 6.1) and the Measurement Guide (figure 6.2) at the front of the notebook, and compare your moles to the illustrations. Always date your notes and be diligent in recording exact numbers of moles and exact sizes.

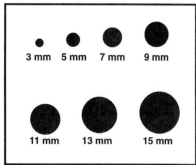

figure 6.2: Measurement Guide

The increase in the number of diagnosed skin cancers coincides with the trend toward spending more time in the sun.

How to Perform a Body Check

Start by having a bath or shower to remove any soil or smudges that may cause confusion. The actual exam will take only about ten minutes. When you give the exam to someone else, follow the same procedure, since consistency promotes accuracy. Take notes of any markings.

1. Start with the easiest areas to examine: your face (especially the nose), arms, and hands (including fingernails and between the fingers). Raise your arms and use the mirror to examine the backs of your upper arms (including underarms). Make notes.

2. Then work from the top down. Using the blow-dryer and a comb, make parts through your hair—one row at a time—over the top of your head and down to your ears to check for any lesion covered by hair. You can check the back of your head using a handheld mirror, but this is cumbersome. Ask someone to help. Make notes.

3. With your back to the full-length mirror, use the handheld mirror to check your neck (front and back), shoulders, chest, and torso. Check the upper back and sides. Women should check the undersides of the breasts. You may want to use a checklist so you don't forget any area.

4. Still using both mirrors, check your lower back, backs of both legs, and buttocks.

5. Sit down, prop each leg in turn on the other chair and check the front and sides of both legs (thigh to shin), ankles, the tops of the feet, between the toes, and under the toenails. Examine the heels and soles of

The sun's circumference is 2.7 million miles.

feet. Again, even if you have not found anything suspicious, use a checklist so that you know you have covered everything.

6.   Still sitting, again prop each leg in turn on the other chair and use the handheld mirror to examine the genitals.

Once you complete the entire body check, be sure that you correctly enter all information in your notebook *with a date*. This is especially important for those at high risk for melanoma, those who are monitoring changes for a doctor, and those who are helping to monitor others.

Body Checks by a Doctor

Not all doctors are well versed in spotting melanoma. However, most can identify lesions that look suspicious and can track changes in your skin. If you are in a high risk category, your general practitioner may refer you to a specialist. Further, you should not hesitate to ask to be referred to a specialist if you have any concerns.

Many dermatologists offer free skin cancer screenings through the AAD and The Skin Cancer Foundation. It is easy to find out when and where these are held by looking at the organization's Web site or by calling them (see "Online Resources"). Generally, these screenings are held in the spring or early summer in an effort to remind people to use sun protection. However, if you find a suspicious change on your skin, call your doctor and make an immediate appointment. Do not wait until the next free screening.

If you are at high risk for melanoma, we encourage you to have an annual screening done by an expert even if you give yourself periodic self-exams.

The sun is 109 times larger than the earth.

. . . .

What to Do If You Think You Might Have Melanoma

If you find something growing on your skin that you think might be a melanoma, don't procrastinate and don't panic. Most lesions and changes in pigmentation are not cancerous, but timing is crucial in treating melanomas. Call your doctor immediately and make an appointment. Often, because of insurance requirements, you will need to see your general practitioner or your primary care physician for a referral to a specialist, usually a dermatologist.

Remember, throughout the process of finding out what you have and how it should be treated, you must be your own advocate. Doctors can and do make mistakes, and not all doctors are familiar enough with melanoma symptoms to make a correct diagnosis. Your primary care physician might decide to perform a biopsy before referring you, which would confirm whether or not the lesion or change is in fact cancerous. If, however, your doctor does not do a biopsy and says just to watch the spot for six months, make sure that you are convinced that the doctor knows what the lesion is and how it should progress during those six months. If the doctor does not know, or if the lesion does not progress as the doctor said it should during the first week or two, insist that it be checked sooner and ask for a referral to a specialist, preferably a dermatologist. If your gut feeling tells you that you have something that should be checked further, make sure that it is.

Once you have a referral to a dermatologist, be sure to tell the person making appointments that you think you have a suspicious mole or skin change. Given that information, most dermatologists will try to see you immediately. Many dermatologists, particularly those with practices in the Sun Belt states, leave time at the end of the day to see possible new melanoma cases. Unfortunately, as the number of skin cancer cases increases, as will happen over the next decade, you may need to call more than one dermatologist to get an appointment. Be persistent. However, remember that most changes in the skin are not melanoma and that when detected and treated early, melanoma can be removed with excellent cure rates.

The sun is about 4.5 billion years old.

Diagnosis

A biopsy is the only way to make a definite diagnosis. As we discussed in the last chapter, most biopsies are relatively minor, office-based procedures that require only local anesthesia. The doctor will usually try to remove all of the suspicious-looking growth as part of the biopsy. This is called an *excisional biopsy.*

Excisional surgery or biopsy is widely used to treat all kinds of skin cancer. The surgeon outlines the tumor with a safety margin of healthy-looking tissue, injects a local anesthetic, waits until the area is numb, removes both the tumor and the healthy tissue immediately surrounding it, then stitches the area. The entire procedure is quick and easy, and the wound usually heals within a week to ten days. If the growth is too large to be removed entirely, the doctor takes a sample of the tissue.

The tissue specimen is sent to a laboratory, where a *pathologist,* or specially trained physician, examines the tissue under a microscope to check for cancer cells. While this sounds simple, this is the most crucial step in determining the correct treatment if any further treatment is needed. The pathologist will determine if any cancerous cells are present and if they have invaded the surrounding tissue.

If the report says that the specimen is hard to interpret, do not assume there is no cancer. Ask that it be reviewed by a *dermatopathologist* (a specialist in the pathology of skin) or by a pathologist specializing in dermatology. Or simply ask for a second opinion.

Further, be sure to ask for a copy of the pathology report. It is always a good idea to have accurate records for future reference, and the report will be particularly useful if you decide to get a second opinion.

If the report says that the cancer has exceeded the borders of the lesion, it is assumed that the cancer is still present in the patient. Your doctor will need to know what stage the cancer is in before proceeding.

The sun will remain more or less the way it is for another 5 billion years.

Staging

Staging provides a guideline for treatment based on how far the disease has spread. The doctor measures how thick the tumor is, or how deeply the melanoma has invaded the skin, and will check whether melanoma cells have spread to nearby lymph nodes or to other parts of the body. Based on the doctor's findings, a stage number will be assigned to the melanoma, indicating a general prognosis.

Stage 0. When melanoma cells are found only in the epidermis or top layer of the skin and have not invaded deeper tissues, it can be easily removed with an extremely high cure rate. However, even if you have had only stage 0 melanoma, you should be aware that you are in a high risk category for another melanoma. You should perform routine checks for the rest of your life and alert your family that they too may be at risk.

Stage I. The tumor is no more than one millimeter (one twenty-fifth of an inch) thick and the top layer of skin may appear scraped or ulcerating, or the tumor is between one and two millimeters (one-twelfth of an inch) and there is no ulceration. The melanoma cells have not spread to nearby lymph nodes, and like stage 0 melanoma, it can be easily removed with a high cure rate. Again, however, if you have had stage 1 melanoma, you are at a high risk of developing another.

Stage II. The tumor is at least one millimeter thick. It may be between one and two millimeters thick with ulceration, or it is more than two millimeters with possible ulceration. While much thicker than stage 0 or I, the melanoma cells in stage II have not spread to nearby lymph nodes. This means that it can be easily removed and the five-year survival rate is still high.

Stage III. The melanoma cells have grown deeply into the skin and have spread to nearby tissues. They may or may not have spread to one or more nearby lymph nodes. It can still be removed, but cure is more difficult.

The earth is about 4.5 billion years old.

Stage IV. The melanoma cells have spread to other organs, to lymph nodes, or to areas far away from the original tumor. This stage has a poor survival rate.

According to the American Cancer Society, the five-year survival rate for melanoma in stages 0, I, and II is 96 percent; survival rates for stages III and IV are 60 and 14 percent respectively. About 82 percent of melanomas are diagnosed in stages 0, I, and II (ACS 2004b). African-Americans diagnosed with melanoma have an overall five-year survival rate of only 58.8 percent, compared with 84.8 percent for Caucasians, because the disease is typically detected at later stages (Byrd et al. 2004).

Questions to Ask

Remember, you must be your own advocate. Doctors will do everything they can to help you, but this can be a complicated disease and you can help fight it by being informed.

Often, particularly at cancer centers, a team of specialists will work together to treat melanoma. The team may include a dermatologist, surgeon, oncologist, radiation oncologist, and plastic surgeon. You can trust these doctors, but you may have questions and concerns they have not addressed with you. Feel free to ask any doctor treating you about any concern you may have. Bring a notepad or a tape recorder with you to appointments and write down your questions ahead of time. These can be stressful conversations, and you won't want to forget any of your questions. Further, you may want to check your doctor's credentials. This is not difficult. The American Board of Medical Specialties provides an online list of doctors' names along with their specialty and educational background (see "Online Resources").

Do not worry if you don't think of all your questions at once. Your doctors will likely be available to answer questions as you proceed. You can find lists of questions you may want to ask through The Skin Cancer Foundation, the AAD, the National Cancer Institute, and the Melanoma International Foundation (see "Online Resources").

The sun is 93 million miles away from the earth.

Treatments

Treatments for melanoma usually include surgery, chemotherapy, biological therapy, or radiation therapy. Some cases require a combination of treatments; others respond to one. Clinical trials or research studies may provide more treatment options. Talk to your doctor to find out what these involve and how they can affect your treatment.

Surgery

Surgery is the preferred treatment for melanoma because it is the fastest and surest way to rid your skin of the cancer. The doctor removes the tumor and some of the surrounding tissue, making sure all cancerous cells are taken. The amount of surrounding skin that is removed depends on the thickness of the melanoma and how deeply it has invaded the layers of the skin.

If a large area of skin has to be removed in a cosmetically sensitive area, such as the face or neck, a *skin graft* is used. Skin from another part of the body is used to replace the skin that was removed at the site of the melanoma.

Sentinel lymph node biopsy. Using a radioactive substance to create images of the lymph nodes, a surgeon can trace the pathway that the melanoma is taking from the tumor by highlighting the first lymph node it has entered. That node is then removed by the surgeon and examined under the microscope by a pathologist, who determines if cancerous cells are present. If this first node or *sentinel node* contains cancer cells, the surgeon removes the rest of the lymph nodes in the area. If it does not contain cancer cells, no additional lymph nodes are removed.

Lymph node dissection. In *lymph node dissection,* the surgeon removes all the *regional nodes,* or lymph nodes in the area of the melanoma. This is done in an effort to keep the cancer from spreading throughout the body. On average, 40 to 50 percent of people with regional node involvement are cured. The overall range is 15 to 70

The core temperature of the sun is roughly 10 million degrees Fahrenheit.

percent, depending on the number of lymph nodes involved and other factors (Poole and Guerry 1998).

Nonsurgical Treatments

If melanoma has spread to other parts of the body, surgery alone is no longer an effective treatment. Several nonsurgical treatments are available. If it seems likely that the melanoma has spread, *adjuvant therapy* may be used. This therapy is designed to eliminate cancerous cells that may have escaped the primary tumor or lymph nodes before they were removed.

Alpha interferon. *Alpha interferon* is approved by the Food and Drug Administration (FDA) as adjuvant therapy for melanoma patients. It is a synthetic protein identical to the protein the body creates to fight viral infections. Studies have shown fairly good success rates for five-year periods when patients use alpha interferon (Kirkwood et al. 1996). However, it is important to know that this is an expensive treatment with many difficult side effects. Using alpha interferon is a decision you must make carefully with your doctor.

Biological therapy. Also called *immunotherapy,* biological therapy uses the body's own immune system to fight the melanoma. An example of this type of therapy is an experimental vaccine that is derived from the patient's own melanoma. (These vaccines have not yet been proved effective, nor have they been approved, and they are usually reserved for patients who have metastasized melanoma or are at a high risk of recurrence.) Other new therapies that stimulate the immune system to attack melanoma are also being researched.

Chemotherapy. *Chemotherapy* is the use of powerful drugs to kill cancer cells. The drugs are given in cycles. For example, you may be given medication by mouth or by injection for the first five days of the month for six months. The drugs enter the bloodstream and travel throughout the body. There are always side effects. Find out what they are in advance and ask your doctor for methods to help you cope. Most chemotherapy drugs make you especially sensitive to the sun,

The surface temperature of the sun is roughly 5,800 degrees Fahrenheit.

and you should be extremely careful to avoid UVR exposure or to use effective sun protection methods.

In *isolated limb perfusion*, these same powerful drugs are injected directly into the limb that has melanoma. The flow of blood to and from that limb is stopped for a short while, allowing the drug to reach the tumor directly and destroy the cancerous cells.

Radiation therapy. Radiation therapy uses high-energy rays to kill cancer cells. It is usually used to help control melanoma that has spread to the brain, bones, and other parts of the body. It may shrink tumors and relieve symptoms.

Other Treatments to Consider

Acting as your own advocate, you should find out all you can about different treatments. This is equally important regardless of the stage of your melanoma. If you have stage III or IV melanoma, you will want to know that all options are being considered.

Clinical trials. There are no uniform standards in treating widespread, metastasized melanoma (stages III and IV). A clinical trial is one way to try an experimental treatment under a doctor's supervision. There are, however, some requirements for these programs. Generally, you must be over eighteen, and you can't be too sick. If the melanoma has spread to certain areas, you may not qualify. Talk to your doctor about these trials or find out about them through the National Cancer Institute.

Alternative medicines. Medicines or remedies that have not been approved by the FDA are generally termed "alternative." Most doctors will not recommend them, because there is little or no research to support claims of success. If you decide to try alternative medicine, discuss it with your doctor, since it may conflict with your current therapy.

Nutrition. Good nutrition helps people fighting cancer to maintain their energy and spirits. The National Cancer Institute (2003a) encourages cancer patients to talk to their doctors and dietitians to find ways to maintain a healthy diet. They also provide a booklet,

UVB radiation is known to cause sunburn.

"Eating Hints for Cancer Patients," which contains many useful ideas and recipes (see "Online Resources").

Life after Melanoma

Melanoma changes your life. For some, the acute awareness that they are vulnerable to a potentially fatal disease is overwhelming. For others, coping with the daily practicalities of treating the disease is monumental. Support groups are available and highly recommended. The Cancer Information Service (see "Online Resources") helps patients and their families locate programs and services.

Remember, once you have had a melanoma, you are at high risk of developing another. Therefore, follow-up care is essential. This should include regular checkups with your doctor and periodic self-exams. Your doctor should give you a schedule indicating when to have checkups. If you had a thick melanoma or it spread to other tissues, your follow-up exams may include blood tests, X-rays, and other scans.

Summing Up

Melanoma is deadly, and the incidence of melanoma in this country is on the rise. If you are at risk for this disease, give yourself routine body checks for any suspicious change in a mole or elsewhere on your skin. Remember that cure rates are high with early treatment. If you find a suspicious change, make an immediate appointment with a doctor. Remember to alert your family if they are at risk.

Help prevent melanoma by being AWARE. Use sun protection every day. For more information, see "Online Resources" at the end of the book.

Only twenty minutes of sun exposure can cause skin damage.

✳ PART II ✳

who needs sun protection?

* 7 *

factors that determine your sensitivity to the sun

How do you know if you are likely to get skin cancer? How do you determine if you are sun sensitive and need sun protection more than your friends need it? Some people need to be extremely aware of protecting themselves, while others can be more relaxed. You should know your individual risk factors and act accordingly. The degree to which you need to protect yourself from the sun depends on your skin type, your health history, and how much time you spend outdoors. In this chapter, we'll take a look at the first two factors.

. . . .
Skin Type

Pathak, Jimbow, and Fitzpatrick (1976) developed a system for classifying skin based on a person's response to about one hour of sun exposure after a winter season in the northern latitudes, or the degree to which a person will burn or tan. Skin types are ranked from type I (most sun sensitive, or most likely to be damaged by sun exposure) to type VI (least likely to experience sun damage). As we discussed in chapter 3, the amount of melanin or pigmentation in your skin is a strong indicator of whether you are sensitive to the sun.

Dermatologists recommend that you know your skin type so that you can use it as a guide for sun protection. Use the following guidelines to determine which skin type you are:

I   Always burns easily, never tans (pale white skin, blue or hazel eyes, freckles, blond or red hair)

II   Usually burns easily, tans minimally with difficulty after repeated exposures (white skin; blond, red, or brown hair; blue, green, or hazel eyes)

III   Sometimes burns moderately, tans moderately and uniformly (white to olive skin). This is the largest group in the United States

IV   Burns minimally, tans profusely and shows immediate tanning reaction (olive or light brown skin, dark brown hair, dark eyes)

V   Very rarely burns but tans profusely (dark brown skin)

VI   Never burns (very dark brown/black skin or deeply pigmented skin)

While the skin type chart is used by most dermatologists, some conclusions that were drawn from it in the 1970s have since changed. For example, if your skin is type IV, V, or VI and you tan easily or never burn, you may think your skin provides all the protection you need. This is not correct. It is true that people with dark skin get fewer skin cancers than people with fair skin, but people of all colors can get skin cancer. No one is immune to the damage that can be caused by UVR. Everyone needs some level of protection, although individuals with type I, II, or III skin have a higher risk of skin cancer. Lack of knowledge in the past about skin types and the effects of UVR allowed people to develop a dangerous lifestyle: tanning for fashion and outdoor leisure activities without sun protection. The

UVC kills bacteria.

increase in skin cancer is a result of this lifestyle. Changing your life-style and using sun protection will help decrease your risk of skin cancer.

Skin Types I and II

If you think about skin type in terms of SPF, a skin type of I or II has an SPF of less than 1, which is barely measurable (Pathak 1999). Melanomas are found most often in this group because they have little pigmentation and therefore almost no defense against UVR. The amount of damage that is caused by UVR exposure will depend on the UVR dose absorbed by the skin. In these two skin types, the damage affects both the epidermal and dermal cells, includ-ing the keratinocytes, melanocytes, Langerhans cells, *endothelial cells* (cells lining the organs of circulation), and *fibroblasts* (cells of connec-tive tissue). Every layer of the skin is damaged, potentially setting off the reaction needed to initiate skin cancer. Skin types I and II need constant and effective sun protection.

People in this group are generally of Celtic, Scandinavian, or northern European descent. Numerous studies over the years have tried to determine why light-skinned people are generally found fur-ther from the equator and dark-skinned people are found closer to it. While the studies are inconclusive, one theme that emerges is that heavier pigmentation found in populations closer to the equator may be an evolutionary form of protection against too much sun and dis-eases such as melanoma. The lower pigmentation in populations far from the equator may be an evolutionary response to enhance vita-min D production and prevent diseases such as rickets.

This may also help explain why there has been a rise in the number of skin cancers seen among light-skinned people. In Austra-lia, the light-skinned people who had moved there from the British Isles were necessarily unprotected (except by clothing)—unlike the very dark Aboriginal people—and as a result of the fashion changes during the thirties, forties, and fifties, skin cancers became prevalent beginning in the nineteen-seventies. In America, a similar dynamic is taking place now.

UVR was added to the National Institutes of Health
list of carcinogens in 2000.

Skin Type III

People with a skin type of III are naturally lightly pigmented and tan more evenly than people with skin types I or II when exposed to the sun. The average Caucasian is a skin type III. When a person with this skin type gets tanned, there is an increase in melanin pigmentation of the skin, which offers a little protection from DNA damage. However, the protection is minimal—less than SPF 2. You cannot tan unless you damage the epidermal cells. Tans are also considered an immediate sign of photodamage, which may not be obvious until later but is mostly irreversible.

Skin Types IV, V, and VI

People with skin types IV, V, and VI can produce a tan with less DNA damage than skin types I, II, and III. Types IV and V typically include descendants of Italians, Spaniards, and Greeks; type V includes descendants of Asians and many Hispanics; and type VI includes descendants of black Africans. But since these groups have merged over the years, there is no standard for ethnic skin colors. Many African-Americans have light skin, while descendants from northern Europe can have dark skin.

The increased melanin of a tan in skin types IV, V, and VI may offer a little protection against subsequent UVR exposure. However, even with this increased pigmentation, there is no full protection against the harm caused by UVR. For example, a base tan in a person with type IV skin may provide an SPF of only 2 to 2.5 (Pathak 2002).

As we mentioned in chapter 6, skin cancers—particularly melanoma—in dark-skinned people are also increasing but are often diagnosed at a later and more dangerous stage. Perhaps the increase is due to the fact that over the past few decades, more dark-skinned people, like white-skinned people, have followed trends and exposed their unprotected skin to UVR. Possibly there is also a correlation to the depleted ozone layer and global warming. The fact that these diagnoses are being made at a later and more dangerous stage is more likely a result of a lack of education about skin cancers among dark-skinned people.

UVR is the main cause of most skin cancers.

Whatever the reason for the increased number of melanoma and nonmelanoma skin cancers among people of all colors, our best advice is to enjoy the natural color of your skin and protect it from changing. If you think of your skin type in terms of the SPF it provides, you will agree that everyone needs some protection and it is particularly important for those people with skin types I, II, and III.

Medical History

The risk factors for developing skin cancers go beyond skin color. One of the most telling risks is whether there is a pattern of skin cancer in your immediate (blood) family. This can be determined with a medical history.

The term "medical history" can be confusing. Does it mean individual medical history, or does it mean family medical history? It means both. Your own medical history is more easily understood when put in the context of a family history. However, do not be lured into thinking that if there is no history of skin cancer in your family, you won't get it. Nor should you be overly alarmed if someone in your family has had skin cancer. Simply be aware of the facts—if you don't know, find out if anyone in your blood family has had melanoma or other skin cancers—and tell your doctor.

Genetic Risk

There is no doubt that a genetic connection exists in melanoma-prone families. These are families where the melanoma patient has two blood relatives who have melanoma. Some of the connections are obvious, such as skin type and numbers of moles. Others, such as a possible mutant gene, are being researched. Eventually, genetic testing may be available for susceptibility to melanoma, as it is for breast and colon cancer. In the meantime, studies show that between 5 and 10 percent of people who develop melanoma have a close family member with the disease (Masci and Borden 2002). Furthermore, if any of your family members have had basal or

Sunburns and tans are forms of phototrauma.

squamous cell cancer, you have an increased risk of developing a similar cancer or melanoma (ACS 2003).

People at risk of developing malignant melanoma generally fall into one of two groups. The first is sun-sensitive Caucasians (skin types I and II—people of Irish, Scottish, Norwegian, or Celtic descent). The second group includes people who have a family history of malignant melanomas and have inherited the gene that places them at increased risk. They tend to develop a number of moles (Tucker et al. 1997). Moles that change are not always in obvious places, like the forearms or face. You may find them on the back of your neck or on your scalp or shoulders. Pigmented birthmarks can also change and become melanomas.

If you have a lot of moles, whether they are dysplastic or ordinary, you are more susceptible to melanoma than the average person. This is generally an inherited trait, and is considered a marker identifying people who are at an increased risk of developing melanoma at the site of the mole or elsewhere on the body.

A person who has dysplastic moles and a personal or family history of melanoma is thought to have a high risk of developing melanoma (Tucker et al. 1997). However, remember that melanoma detected and treated early is almost always curable. Be sure to periodically check your whole body for any changes to the skin (see chapter 6) and always use sun protection. The Skin Cancer Foundation also recommends a regular checkup (at least once a year) from a physician who specializes in skin disease (SCF 2003b).

Burns

Burns, regardless of their cause, can badly damage skin and leave it sun sensitive. This is true for any skin type.

Diseases or Skin Conditions

There are several skin conditions that are immediately and adversely affected by exposure to UVR. These are part of the medical history of the person who has the disease and should be reported by

For every 1 percent decrease in the ozone layer, there can be an increase of up to 3 percent in skin cancer rates (Scotto 1986)

blood relatives as part of their family medical history. We have listed a few of these diseases below, but if you are ever diagnosed with a skin disease or disorder, you should ask whether it is sensitive to UVR.

Lupus. This is a multisystem disease with a tendency to cause *photo-sensitive* (caused by an abnormal reaction to UVR) skin rashes. Almost 1.5 million Americans suffer from lupus (Lupus Foundation 2004), and nearly 80 percent get sun-induced rashes or complain of sun-related problems (Lupus UK 2004). Further, lupus is often caused or aggravated by sun exposure. Research shows that among Caucasians, prolonged sun exposure causes a threefold increase in the chance of developing lupus (Fraser et al. 2003).

Multiple sclerosis. This is a chronic autoimmune disorder affecting movement, sensation, and bodily functions. It is caused by destruction of the *myelin* insulation covering nerve fibers *(neurons)* in the central nervous system (brain and spinal cord). Multiple sclerosis affects more than 400,000 Americans and more than 2 million people worldwide (NMSS 2004). Symptoms of multiple sclerosis may be worsened by sun exposure, and patients are warned to stay out of the sun. Further, many drugs prescribed for multiple sclerosis cause sun sensitivity (especially interferon beta-1a).

Sjögren's syndrome. This is a chronic disease in which white blood cells attack the moisture-producing glands, including sweat glands. The hallmark symptoms are dry eyes and dry mouth, but it is a systemic disease affecting many organs. As many as 4 million Americans have this disease (Sjögren's Syndrome Foundation 2004). People with Sjögren's syndrome must protect their eyes and skin from the drying effects of UVR.

Albinism. If you are born with *albinism,* or partial or total lack of melanin (the pigment produced by the melanocytes in the epidermis), exposure to UVR will cause severe sunburn, skin inflammations or rashes, and skin cancer. Albinism is found in all races, and one person in 17,000 in the United States has some form of this disease (NOAH 2002). It is not always recognized, since very fair hair and skin are appropriate for some ethnic backgrounds, but those who have it are

The thickness of the ozone layer changes with the weather.

always sun sensitive. Albinos have pale skin, white hair, and some-times pink eyes.

Vitiligo. This condition can develop in people of any age and pro-duces irregular patches of skin anywhere on the body that lack pig-ment. This disease affects one or two of every one hundred people (AAD 1999b). It is believed to be caused by the immune system work-ing against the melanocytes, stopping the production of melanin or pigment. These patches easily burn when exposed to UVR and need to be protected at all times.

Xeroderma pigmentosum. This is an extremely rare genetic disor-der. It is an inability to repair ultraviolet-damaged DNA and is charac-terized by severe sensitivity to all UVR sources. Those who have xeroderma pigmentosum have a greater than thousandfold increased risk of skin cancer or precancerous tumors (XPS 2004).

Not all diseases that are sensitive to UVR are listed here. If you are not sure, ask your doctor or contact the AAD (see "Online Resources").

. . . .
Medications

Many drugs or medications, such as antibiotics, *psoralens* (substances found in figs, limes, parsnip roots, and other plants that are used in making drugs), and *diuretics* (substances that increase the discharge of urine), can increase the skin's susceptibility to reddening and burning from UVR exposure. These drugs are *photosensitizing agents.* You should always carefully read labels and pay attention to warnings about side effects. Look for warnings like "This product may cause adverse reactions to ultraviolet rays" or "This medicine may cause sensitivity to the sun." If you have any questions, ask your doctor or your pharma-cist. If you take drugs that cause sun sensitivity, use effective sun pro-tection regardless of your skin type.

More specifically, *photosensitivity* is a reaction that occurs when a photosensitizing agent (ingredient in a drug), either in or on the skin,

UVR intensity increases at higher altitudes.

reacts to UVR. This can be caused by both topical and systemic drugs and is classified as either phototoxic or photoallergic.

In a *phototoxic* reaction, the skin reacts as if poisoned, exhibiting symptoms shortly after the person uses the medicine. Phototoxic reactions are common and can be produced in most individuals given a high enough dose of the drug and sufficient UVR exposure. The reaction usually occurs within five to twenty hours and resembles an exaggerated sunburn. It is confined to areas exposed to UVR. People using these drugs should avoid direct sunlight and use sun protection.

Photoallergic reactions occur in individuals who have been previously sensitized to UVR and are predisposed to have a reaction. The reaction may take up to twenty-four hours to occur, and symptoms will occur all over the body, not just on exposed areas.

These two types of photosensitivity are caused by sulfa drugs and some other antibiotics. Some medications that treat acne, blood pressure, constipation, heart disease, diabetes, fluid retention, psychiatric disorders, bladder or kidney infection, cancer, and colds can cause UVR sensitivity. The medicines you take internally may cause an overall adverse reaction whenever you are exposed to UVR, while topical medications will likely only cause problems at the specific area.

Some drugs used for chemotherapy to treat cancer are photosensitizers. Talk to your doctor about them. They can cause severe reactions when the user is exposed to UVR.

Not all people who use drugs that cause photosensitivity will be affected. It is important to know the potential problems associated with any medications you take so you can protect yourself accordingly. See "Online Resources" at the end of the book for reputable sources that list drugs that cause sun sensitivity.

Surgery

People who have had surgery are usually sun sensitive and therefore likely to burn, potentially triggering skin cancers. There are several different reasons for this, the most important yet least obvious being that the drugs given after surgery to fight infections are photosensitizers. If possible, ask your doctor before surgery about any medications you will be given.

The area that receives the most UVR is the equator.

At the site of the surgery, scar tissue forms that lacks the same levels of melanin as normal skin. This lower level of melanin will not increase over time, and even the smallest scar will burn, turning a bright pink. Scars can become the sites of skin cancers.

If you have had surgery and are taking medications, or if you have scarring anywhere on exposed skin, be AWARE of the need to protect yourself from UVR exposure.

Summing Up

Many different factors determine whether you are sun sensitive. Become AWARE of your need for sun protection by learning your skin type, knowing your individual and family medical history, and checking all medications for sun sensitivity warnings. Everyone, regardless of color, is sun sensitive to some degree.

UVR is most intense at noon.

children need sun protection and education

It's wonderful to see your children playing outside. Swings, sandboxes, bicycles, roller skates, jump ropes, pools, puddles, and melting ice-cream cones are ingredients for a happy childhood. However, children should be taught from an early age to be AWARE of the problems associated with sun exposure and the need to use sun protection. In this chapter, we'll look at the reasons children need sun protection and discuss the best approaches to sun protection for children from birth through the teenage years.

Exposure During Childhood May Cause Skin Cancers Later

For most children, 23 percent of their lifetime UVR exposure will happen before the age of eighteen (Godar et al. 2003). While 23 percent is not as high as the widely quoted figure of 80 percent (now shown to be a misinterpretation), the damage is significant and can be compounded by subsequent exposure.

Stern, Weinstein, and Baker (1986) developed a model from which an assumption was made that using a sunscreen with an SPF of 15 or higher on children under eighteen would reduce nonmelanoma skin cancer later in life by 78 percent. This showed that if the initial damage in childhood can be prevented, later problems may be avoided, and this model was consistent with other findings. For example, Cooke and Fraser (1985) showed that lower numbers of skin cancers were diagnosed among fair-skinned people who arrived in Australia after the age of fifteen compared with those of similar descent who were born and spent their childhood in Australia. Studies in California showed a similar outcome. People who had migrated to the state after the age of fifteen from areas where the sun was less intense developed fewer and less serious skin cancers later in life than people who had grown up in the state (Mack and Floderus 1991). From these studies, Godar (2001) draws the conclusion that the most important factors contributing to melanoma are exposure to UVR in early childhood, sunburns, and intermittent exposure to UVR. These three factors, along with cumulative exposure, also play a role in nonmelanoma skin cancers.

To try to fully address the concerns about childhood exposures, experts around the world are beginning to question whether protection advice should take location (latitude) into account. However, given that many fair-skinned children live far from the equator and receive intense, often intermittent UVR exposure from many sources (including reflection by snow or water), and given that more skin cancers are being diagnosed in people of color, we believe all children—regardless of their skin color or where they live—should follow the AWARE methods of sun protection every day.

. . . .
What about Vitamin D?

Some parents are concerned that if their children are protected from the sun, they won't produce enough vitamin D. This is a valid concern, because vitamin D, also known as the "sunshine vitamin," is

The UV index is often displayed with your local weather.

essential for strong bones and calcium absorption. However, Hurwitz (1988) found that only a few minutes of exposure to UVR, two to three times a week, is sufficient for adequate vitamin D production.

The American Academy of Pediatrics has also addressed this issue and recommends that all healthy infants from two months old, children, and adolescents receive 200 IU of vitamin D per day (Gartner and Greer 2003). Infant formulas and cow's milk are fortified with vitamin D at these levels. Vitamin D supplements, in drop or tablet form, are available over the counter as part of multivitamin preparations. Ask your pediatrician if they are needed and be careful not to give too much vitamin D because high doses can be toxic.

The Cancer Council of Australia (2003) does advise that there are segments of the population that may be at risk of vitamin D deficiency. These include the elderly, the infirm, people who don't go outdoors, dark-skinned people who cover their skin for cultural reasons, and very young or premature babies. It is generally advised that these people boost vitamin D intake through diet or supplements.

Sensible sun protection should not put you or your children at risk of vitamin D deficiency.

. . . .

Sun Protection for Children

For the past twenty years, sunscreen has been the primary sun protection method used for children. In 1997 the AAD found that as many as 74 percent of parents reported using some form of sun protection for their children, with 53 percent using sunscreen. The survey findings also indicated there had been an increase in awareness among adults that sun exposure is dangerous and a decline in the belief that having a tan is healthy (CDC 1998). Unfortunately, this awareness appears to now have less impact. A study by Johnson and colleagues (2001) in Florida found that only 33 percent of parents used any form of protection for their children and that sunscreen alone was the method most commonly used. Further, the study showed that the children spent a substantial amount of time outdoors (between one and five hours a day) and that parents believed it was okay for children to stay out in the sun longer if they wore sunscreen—a behavior associated with the

Top shade alone will not block all UVR.

subsequent development of greater numbers of moles. Other recent studies have shown that sunscreen is not applied often enough to be effective (sunscreen needs to be reapplied every two hours), that not enough is applied, and that children often rub or wash it off (Wright, Wright, and Wagner 2001). These studies illustrate the need for continuous education and show why children need other methods of sun protection—clothing, shade, and avoidance—despite the large percentage of parents who apply sunscreen.

The American Academy of Pediatrics now advises against using sunscreen alone to protect children from UVR exposure (AAPCEH 1999). Children should be protected from exposure to UVR by using sunscreen combined with sun protection clothing, hats, sunglasses, avoidance, and shade. The following sections will discuss the best methods of protection offered for each age group. Children are never too young or too old to learn the importance of sun protection.

How to Protect Your Baby from the Sun

Babies' skin is extremely sensitive and can burn easily. A combination of sun protection methods should be used from their very first day and continued throughout their lives. These methods are slightly different from sun protection methods for older children, but used consistently, they will help form beneficial lifelong habits.

The Australian SunSmart program, the AAD, The Skin Cancer Foundation, and the Environmental Protection Agency recommend similar strategies for protecting babies from UVR.

Avoid Peak UV Times

Start a daily habit of checking the UV index for the area where you live. The National Weather Service and the Environmental Protection Agency both provide a daily UV index, which predicts peak UVR times for the following day. Based on this forecast, you can organize your day to avoid exposing your baby to direct sunlight during the peak UV times. For example, you can take your baby for a

Tanning beds cause skin cancer.

walk early in the morning or late in the afternoon and plan indoor activities or activities in the shade for the middle of the day.

Cover Your Baby's Skin

Dress your baby in loose-fitting outfits that cover arms and legs. Baby outfits made from sun protective material—material tested for an *ultraviolet protection factor* (UPF) rating of 30 or higher—are the best protection (chapter 12 provides detailed information about sun protective clothing). Clothing made with natural fibers and a tight weave can be used as an alternative but does not offer guaranteed protection. For example, a T-shirt may provide an SPF of only 5 to 10. If a material is transparent, it does not offer adequate sun protection. Always make sure your baby is not too hot.

Choose a hat that protects the baby's face, neck, and ears, such as a soft legionnaire-style hat, with a flap at the back that will crumple easily when your baby leans back. This will protect the back of your baby's neck and ears. It also provides better cover for the side of your baby's face. A baby who wears a hat during the first few months will get used to having it on and as a toddler will be less likely to resist wearing it.

Sunglasses are not very practical for a young baby. However, your baby's eyes can be damaged by UVR exposure. To protect your baby's eyes, stay out of the sun during peak UV times, put a hat on your baby, and keep your baby in the shade.

Seek Shade

Babies are at risk for sunburn even when they are in the shade. UVR is reflected onto the skin from surfaces such as buildings, concrete, sand, and water. There are many different types of structures that you can purchase to add shade to your backyard or patio or take with you to the beach. Umbrellas, tents, cabanas, lean-tos, and some stretched materials all provide shade. The best shade is provided by structures with sides. In chapter 15, we'll discuss these devices and others in more detail. Seek out shade, but be sure to use other sun protection methods as well.

During the eighteenth and nineteenth centuries, members of the royal court in France would powder their faces to look pale.

Choose the Right Sunscreen for Your Baby

Infants under six months of age should be kept out of direct sun and covered by protective clothing. However, if exposure does occur, the American Academy of Pediatrics (2004) and the Cancer Council Australia (2002) recommend using sunscreen on the small areas of the baby's body that are not already covered by a hat and clothing. There is no evidence that using sunscreen on infants is harmful (Marks 1996).

Always test the sunscreen on a small area of the baby's skin the first time you use it. If there is any skin reaction—such as a rash, reddening, or spots—wash it off and do not use it. Try other sunscreens until you find one that does not cause a reaction. We recommend that you use a sunscreen with an SPF of 30 or higher. Sunscreen should be applied twenty minutes before going outdoors and reapplied every two hours, or more often if it has been wiped or rubbed off. Do not use a sunscreen that is past its use-by date or does not have a use-by date.

Around Town with Your Baby

It doesn't take much to develop habits that will help protect your baby from UVR exposure. It does, however, require some planning ahead.

Pack a baby bag and leave it ready for any outing. Most parents carry some kind of baby bag when going shopping, visiting, or even jogging. It is easy to keep sun protection items in the bag, and this is a good habit. It is also a good idea to make a checklist. Include the following items, and you will be ready to protect your baby:

* a baby blanket or sheet

* a light shawl

* a soft hat with an all-around brim

Tanning first became fashionable in the 1920s.

* a baggy jumpsuit that covers legs and arms

* sunscreen

While in the car, shield the baby from direct sunlight coming in through the side window.

When purchasing a stroller, check that the hood can be moved to block out direct sunlight. Keep a small, light sheet in the stroller so it can be draped over the top and sides. Watch closely to make sure the sheet does not drop onto the baby and that the stroller remains well ventilated.

A portable umbrella, beach cabana, or sun tent can be left in the trunk of the car so it is always available for picnics or outdoor visits. A shade structure that includes a roof and sides offers much better protection than a structure with a roof only.

Try to find shady places to sit with the baby when outside, but remember to keep the baby covered up as well. Shade does not always block all UVR.

Sun Protection for Toddlers

The Skin Cancer Foundation says, "It's never too early to teach your children about sun protection. They'll learn by your example, so be their role model, and just like they remind you to buckle up in the car, they'll never let you forget to cover up in the sun" (Ayoub 2004).

Once your babies are on their feet, their whole world *and* your whole world changes. Sun protection will take a little more thought and effort on your part, but habits should develop, and it will become easier as your children grow older. Remember that it is never too early or too late to teach your children how to protect themselves from UVR.

Several different guides have been created to help parents with this teaching process. "The ABCs for Fun in the Sun" from the AAD (2000d) is an easy way to learn sun protection methods and is a good way to talk about sun protection with all your child's caregivers.

Gabrielle (Coco) Chanel introduced tanning as fashion.

A = Away   Keep away from direct sunlight, especially midday.

B = Block   Use a broad-spectrum sunscreen. The AAD recommends a minimum SPF of 15; we suggest SPF 30 or higher.

C = Cover up Wear sun protection clothing and a hat.

S = Speak out Be an advocate for sun protection with family, friends, teachers, and community leaders.

While this plan simplifies how to think about protection, you will need to work out how to implement it in advance. We've outlined some of the easiest ways to follow the ABCs of sun protection as well as some challenges you may encounter.

A = Away. Before babies can walk, it is relatively easy to keep them out of the midday sun. However, if you have a toddler, it is important to stay away from the sun without adequate protection. Talk to your caregivers and explain that during the peak UVR hours of 10:00 A.M. to 4:00 P.M., it is especially important to avoid exposure or use effective sun protection. This may not be easy if your child is cared for with many other children, but with your help, the caregivers are likely to want to do what they can. Most caregivers truly want to make sure your child is safe.

Check the outdoor area where you child plays to make sure there are adequately shaded areas. If there is no shade, again speak up and explain why it is needed. (Chapter 15 provides information on inexpensive structures that can provide shade in most areas.) If cost is a problem, recruit other parents to contribute.

B = Block. At home, sunscreen is a relatively easy sun protection method to use. You can apply it yourself and be sure it is reapplied throughout the day. Many dermatologists believe sunscreen should be applied every morning before leaving the house. It should always be applied twenty minutes before exposure to the sun. If you keep the sunscreen in the bathroom where your children brush their teeth and help them apply it at the same time each morning, it will become a habit.

A tan results from your skin defending itself against UVR.

Sunscreen must be reapplied after two hours in the sun. This is especially important for sunscreen to be effective, but it can be a difficult task for caregivers.

A further hindrance is that many states have laws requiring parents to give permission for the use of sunscreen, and if the parent's instructions are different from the package instructions, a medical provider's authorization may be required. Until the laws regarding the application of sunscreen are changed, work with your pediatrician and caregiver to provide the best sun protection for your child.

Give your caregiver pamphlets or published information about sun safety. You can contact the AAD for "The ABCs for Fun in the Sun," or The Skin Cancer Foundation for educational material for young children (see "Online Resources").

C = Cover up. The American Academy of Pediatrics now recommends that children wear sun protective clothing—including shirts, hats, and sunglasses—as their primary defense against UVR (AAP 2004). Follow this advice and make sure your child wears a wide-brimmed hat, long-sleeve shirt, and pants during prolonged periods in the sun. Regular clothing will not always provide sun protection. UVR passes through an open weave or light knits. For example, a T-shirt provides an SPF of only 5 to 10.

It may seem contrary to what you think will be most comfortable on a hot, sunny day, but sun protective clothing actually helps children stay cool while blocking out harmful UVR. Sun protective clothing is usually well ventilated and made with material that keeps moisture away from the skin. Some sun protective clothing is for swimming, so it is fast drying.

In Australia, sun protective clothing has become more popular than sunscreen for protecting children. There are many practical reasons for this shift.

* Most sun protective clothing has a UPF of 30 or higher, which means the material is tested and blocks out 97 percent of UVR.

* You only have to buy it once, rather than buying many bottles or tubes of sunscreen.

A dark tan on white skin offers the protection
equivalent of SPF 2 (Pathak 2002).

* You only have to put it on in the morning. It works all day, even if it gets wet.

* It doesn't have a use-by date, so it can be handed down to younger children.

We have included a complete description of sun protective clothing, including a history of how it was developed and information about how to find it, in chapter 12.

When you dress your toddler in sun protective clothing, don't forget to put sunscreen on areas of skin that are still exposed: face, hands, tops of feet, back of neck.

Hats

Hats are an important part of any sun protection strategy for children. Sun protective hats help shield your child's face and eyes from harmful UVR. Wearing hats at an early age will help establish a lifelong habit. Hats should be worn even on cloudy days.

For years, many people believed that the standard baseball cap provided enough protection. To the contrary, baseball caps provide very little protection. Sun protection hats for children should always have a brim at least two and a half inches wide. A bucket-style hat will protect the face, tops of ears, and much of the neck. Sun protection hats for children are best if they are lightweight, easy to wash, and crushable.

Be sure to put your child's name in the hat, and ask caregivers to be sure the hat is worn whenever your child is outside.

Sunglasses

Protecting your children's eyes from UVR is as important as protecting their skin. Like skin cancers, damage to eyes begins at an early age. Chapter 14 provides information about the need to wear sunglasses and discusses the types of damage UVR exposure can cause. Teach your child never to look directly at the sun and to wear sunglasses when outside.

Up to 80 percent of UVR can penetrate light cloud cover (AMF 2004).

Toddlers can and should wear sunglasses. Look for glasses that provide 99.5 percent UVR protection. Close-fitting, wraparound glasses are best because they block the sun from the sides as well as the front. You may want to include a strap so the glasses don't get lost.

How to Protect Your School-Age Child from the Sun

Most of the sun protection methods used for toddlers and young children should be applied to elementary school children:

* Wear sun protective clothing every day, especially if you live in a warm climate.

* Apply broad-spectrum sunscreen to exposed skin.

* Reapply sunscreen after two hours of UVR exposure, and continue to reapply every two hours while exposed.

* Be sure your child wears a hat during recess.

* Teach your child to look for shaded areas in which to play.

* Teach your child to wear sunglasses while outside.

Unfortunately, there are a lot of difficulties for children trying to follow sun protection methods at school. Here are some of the situations where you may need to become an advocate.

Sunscreen is considered a medicine, and your child may need written permission to use it. Some schools also require that the school nurse be present during application. This becomes an enormous inconvenience for both the nurse and the child, and it discourages the correct use of sunscreen. In California, the Billy Foundation worked to

Sun protective clothing is the new approach to sun protection.

change legislation so children can apply their own sunscreen during school hours.

Many states ban wearing hats on the playground. The Billy Foundation also worked to change this legislation in California, where children are now encouraged to wear sun protective hats during recess. In Hawaii, similar legislation has been passed. Notably, in Australia hats are *required* for outside play at school.

Finding shaded areas on the playground is often impossible. Schools have not been given the funding nor the encouragement to make their playgrounds sun safe.

Wearing sunglasses is not allowed in many schools. Again, this is owing to a lack of awareness and education about sun safety.

In states where sun protection practices have not been addressed or encouraged, you may find that you will need a written request from your child's doctor to allow your child to use sun protection methods. This is one of the best examples of why we need a national skin cancer education and detection campaign in this country.

If you want to protect your elementary school child from harmful UVR exposure, you will need to become an advocate. Give your child's teacher and the school administrators information about the importance of sun protection. Get in touch with your state representatives and ask them to work to change any law that interferes with the use of sun protection. Find out how the Billy Foundation worked to change laws in California (see "Online Resources"), and find out how you can help change similar laws in your own state. Make your child's school sun safe.

The Challenges of Protecting Teenagers

The Australian experience has demonstrated that when sun protection methods are introduced in early childhood and made a habit, preteens and teenagers are more likely to continue to use them.

Haze in the atmosphere can increase UVR exposure.

Since the United States is at the very beginning of the learning curve for sun protection, parents may find it especially challenging to protect their children from sun-damaged skin and skin cancers.

Teenagers typically do not limit their time in the sun, nor do they regularly use sunscreens or other methods of sun protection (Johnson et al. 2001). However, the advent of the technological revolution brought televisions, electronic games, and computers into most American homes, so that today teenagers have more incentive to stay indoors. According to Godar (2001), the American adolescent (age thirteen to nineteen) spends the least time outside compared to any other age group.

Unfortunately, many teens have a preference for tanned skin, and this is a stronger behavior inducement than warnings about the dangers of skin cancer. Johnson and colleagues (2001) found that 83 percent of the children surveyed had at least one sunburn during the previous summer, while 36 percent had three or more. Further, 2 million teenagers in the United States regularly use tanning beds (Dellavalle et al. 2003). These findings suggest that teenagers are perhaps receiving a higher percentage of burns—or one-time intense exposures—than other age groups. Education directed at teenagers must specifically target this behavior.

As a parent, you know that telling your teenage children to protect themselves from UVR is like telling them not to drink soda pop. Most teenagers will agree that too much sugar and caffeine is bad for you and then continue to drink it anyway. Don't give up. You can continue to encourage your teenage children to protect themselves from UVR in many ways:

* having an ongoing discussion about the long-term effects of the sun and the risks of using tanning beds

* occasionally giving examples of someone you know who has aged skin or skin cancer

* making sure they see you using sun protection methods every day

Reflections from water can increase how much UVR you are exposed to.

* keeping sunscreen in their bathroom next to the toothpaste to encourage daily use

* letting them choose their own sun protective hats or clothing

* showing them how to choose the most protective sunglasses

* encouraging them to talk to their friends about sun protection or to take a leadership role in their school to introduce sun protection education

The message about sun protection—like the messages about smoking or sex—needs to come from many different sources, with schools in the lead.

High schools have several different areas where methods of sun protection can be easily taught. The most obvious is through sports programs. For example, in 2003 the AAD, the U.S. Soccer Foundation, and the EPA teamed up to promote sun safety through a public awareness initiative entitled "Make Sun Safety Your Goal." Soccer is often played outdoors during peak sun hours, and coaches are in a unique position to make players, parents, and fans aware of sun safety issues.

Teach Teenagers Skin Cancer Detection Methods

While it is still uncommon, more and more teenagers are being diagnosed with melanoma. Melanoma can be cured with early detection and treatment, so it is important for teenagers to know their skin, look for changes, and get help if they suspect a problem. Teach your teenagers the detection methods in chapter 6.

Moles often don't appear until the teenage years, and it is important to keep track of their size, color, and any changes. If a teen has many moles and freckles, your dermatologist should check them periodically.

UVR is generally lower in the winter months, but can still cause skin cancers.

. . . .

Becoming an Advocate for Sun Protection Education

Prevention of sun exposure is the best way to decrease the numbers of diagnosed skin cancers. Exposure during childhood is a probable triggering factor in the development of many of these cancers. When sun protection practices are taught early and consistently, children can decrease their chance of developing skin cancers later in life.

Health messages for children are best taught by parents and by teachers. However, teaching sun protection in schools without support from the media and society at large is teaching in a vacuum. The message may seem important in the classroom, but it will be quickly forgotten or considered unimportant if it is not heard elsewhere. Further, many parents are unaware of the need for sun protection, and they may not be aware of the different methods of protection. Schools can become the starting point to distribute information and teach sun protection, but they need the support of local, state, and national policies to be effective.

Until that support is provided, you can help build a groundswell of concern by contacting any of the organizations listed in the "Sun Protection Education for Children" section of "Online Resources" to get further information about programs for your school, day care, community center, or any place where sun safety should be a vital concern. Some of these organizations are helpful in lobbying state and local authorities and can give you guidelines for how you too can lobby for change.

Sun Protection Education Programs Really Work

In Australia, the anticancer organizations have spent twenty years initiating educational programs about sun protection and skin cancer detection. In this time, they have been able to measure their success in declining numbers of diagnosed melanomas in the under-fifty age group and in declining numbers of deaths from melanoma for people over fifty. Their success illustrates that sun

Snow reflection can double your overall UVR exposure, especially at higher altitudes.

protection and skin cancer detection education is effective. It also shows how policies of sun protection in schools can make a difference in the fight against skin cancer, especially when those policies are combined with constant and consistent media support and with programs such as sponsored sun protective clothing for sports, greater shade in parks and playgrounds, or eliminating tax on sunscreens.

The EPA's SunWise program shows that children have a measurable change in attitude about sun protection after just a few hours of sun protection education. Unfortunately, another study found that only 3 percent of the 412 schools surveyed had a policy with rules or recommendations for students, teachers, staff, or parents designed to improve sun protection (Buller et al. 2002). The study also showed that many school principals were willing to develop such policies but were unaware of skin cancer as a health problem and were unaware of the role that their schools could play in preventing it.

While we are only in the beginning stages of fighting this epidemic, it is clear that overall success in the schools will depend on educating not just children but the general population. Lessons from Australia teach us that changing behavior and attitudes cannot be accomplished in a void. Messages about prevention and detection must come from many different directions:

* the government, to provide credibility to the problem and to fund campaigns to create awareness;

* the media, to raise awareness of the disease and to explain prevention and detection methods;

* the schools, to teach methods of prevention and to provide a safe environment; and

* parents, to teach their children prevention and detection methods and to become advocates within their communities to bring about involvement at every level.

Once parents are aware of the problem of skin cancer and the epidemic rate at which it is growing, they can become advocates for their children and for their children's friends.

In the early spring, temperatures are low, but UVR is especially strong.

At the local level. Parents can help develop sun protection policies within schools that do not necessarily require changes in legislation. These policies can improve shading on the playground, provide sunscreen reminder notes to other parents before outdoor field trips, suggest tips for better protection during recess or at sports events, and create a sun protection guide as a newsletter.

The Centers for Disease Control and Prevention has published specific and detailed guidelines for school programs to prevent skin cancer. These guidelines outline recommendations for sun policy changes, environmental changes, education programs, family involvement, professional development, and evaluation. You can find them on the CDC Web site under "Guidelines for School Programs to Prevent Skin Cancer." Read them, make copies, and give them to your school principal (see "Online Resources").

At the state level. Parents can help change legislation that directly affects sun safety for their children at school or day care. This can include initiating the funding for sun protection education, allowing hats to be worn at recess or during outdoor sporting events, and allowing children to use sunscreens during school hours.

At the national level. Parents can lobby for a national skin cancer prevention campaign similar to the campaigns against smoking and illegal drug use.

A National Policy Backed by Media Coverage Is Key to Success

Countless studies have been made of the success of the campaign against skin cancer in Australia. While there are many variables that made the campaign effective, extensive and continuous coverage by the media appears to be a key factor.

In Australia, the general population did not intuitively understand skin cancer, and long-standing attitudes about the sun had to be changed. The toughest attitude to change, which is the same attitude held in the United States, is that a tan is desirable. The Cancer Council Victoria decided that only a broad cultural change would

Sunscreen should not be used to increase sun exposure time.

even begin to tackle this attitude. They began with a mass media campaign, "Slip, Slop, Slap," which informed the public of the risks of sun exposure and gave people strategies for protecting themselves. In turn, many organizations and institutions felt pressure to adopt sun protection practices, and eventually it became the norm.

In the United States, mass media campaigns have changed attitudes toward smoking and drinking. As with the anticancer campaigns in Australia, when public awareness is created by media exposure of the issue, programs are introduced within the schools and other institutions that can begin to have a lasting effect.

To date, media exposure in the United States about skin cancer has been piecemeal. This reflects the lack of coordination between the institutions and organizations working to fight skin cancer. The biggest lesson we can learn from Australia is that we need one organization—perhaps the National Council on Skin Cancer Prevention—that is able to research behavior and create key messages. This organization must be backed by strong, stable, and supportive organizations that have common goals and complementary capabilities, and can offer strong and consistent research assistance. This central organization can then create a national policy, coordinate consistent education programs, and oversee a media campaign to educate the public about the hazards of UVR and the importance of sun protection and skin cancer detection.

Financing for the organization and the campaign could be accomplished by taxing the use of tanning beds. A 2 percent tax on this $5 billion industry would provide $100 million per year—enough for programs, media exposure, and the administrative cost of collecting the tax.

The protection offered by sunscreen depends on correct application.

Summing Up

We want our children to enjoy the outdoors. We want them to use their muscles, get fresh air, and find pleasure in all the natural wonders of outdoor life. Sun protection is easy. Learn how to protect your children, teach them to be AWARE and protect themselves, and tell others of the importance of sun protection.

UVR exposure accumulates during the day.

outdoor workers need sun protection and education

Try to think of all the outdoor jobs you know: road construction workers, farmers, telephone line workers, lifeguards, forest rangers, carpenters, painters, builders, tree surgeons, street police, park concession workers, park cleaners, gardeners, sanitation workers, postal workers, dockyard and harbor workers, and drivers.

Risks Associated with Working Outdoors

Traditionally, these jobs require employees to be outdoors six hours or more a day, often during the summer months, when UVR is highest. Traditionally, men hold these jobs. And traditionally, these workers have not had education about sun protection nor about skin cancer prevention and detection. For the millions of Americans who work outdoors, the risk of skin cancer is increased as a result of these traditions.

Workers Are Outdoors Six or More Hours a Day

Outdoor workers receive significantly greater cumulative exposure to UVR than indoor workers. Statistics from Australia show that an outdoor worker is exposed to 20 to 30 percent of the total ambient UVR, depending on the time spent outdoors. In contrast, an indoor worker receives 6 percent in summer or 2 to 4 percent generally (Gies and Wright 2003). In America, Godar and colleagues (2001) developed a very similar estimate for indoor workers, calculating that they receive only 3 percent of total ambient UVR. Godar included children, retirees, homemakers, and stay-at-home parents in her definition of indoor workers. So outdoor workers receive up to ten times as much UVR as most other groups of people.

Gies and Wright (2003) also reported the following statistics:

* Classroom teachers received 7 to 11 percent ambient UVR, while physical education teachers received 30 to 50 percent.

* Gardeners received 44 to 85 percent ambient UVR on the chest and 24 percent on the back, whereas physical education teachers and lifeguards had measured exposures of 8 to 9 percent of ambient UVR on the chest.

* Fishermen, landscape workers, and construction workers were found to receive between 2 and 17 percent of ambient UVR levels, and these levels were significantly reduced when workers wore hats and by seasonal variations.

Cumulative exposure to UVR is considered one of the primary risk factors for nonmelanoma skin cancers. Men experience twice the

Even if you don't feel the heat of the sun, you can be sunburned.

rate of basal cell carcinoma and three times the rate of squamous cell carcinoma as women, which is thought to be the result of higher sun exposure (ACS 2004c). These skin cancers are found on sun-exposed areas such as the head, neck, ears, lips, shoulders, legs, and arms. The most common site is the lips. Outdoor workers with type I or II skin develop more skin cancers than indoor workers (Wooley, Buettner, and Lowe 2002).

Other factors related to sun exposure are also prevalent among outdoor workers, further increasing the risk of skin cancers. For example, Wooley, Buettner, and Lowe (2002) found that most outdoor workers had also spent much of their childhood outdoors. It is less common for someone who preferred indoor activities as a child to later become an outdoor worker. Furthermore, outdoor workers tended to prefer an outdoor lifestyle, which means they spend much of their weekend or off-work time outdoors. The exposure to UVR is not only chronic but nearly constant, and skin cancer is only one of many problems resulting from this kind of exposure. Others include premature aging and eye injuries.

Men Are at a Higher Risk Than Women

While we understand that many women hold outdoor jobs, we think it is helpful to look at the construction industry, one of the largest outdoor industries, where the significant majority of positions (91 percent) are held by men (Conlan 2003). Melanoma diagnoses are about 50 percent higher in men than in women, and about 50 percent more men than women die from melanoma. In 2003, 7,600 deaths were attributed to melanoma—4,700 men and 2,900 women. Older Caucasian males have the highest mortality rates from melanoma (AAD 2004c).

Why would the gender of workers in outdoor jobs be considered a risk factor for skin cancer? Wouldn't the risk be just as high for women who work outdoors? Generally, men view their bodies differently than women and, as a consequence, treat them differently. Women tend to take better care of their skin, whether by wearing

Standards for tanning beds have not been updated since 1985.

sunscreens, applying makeup or moisturizers, or keeping it covered. Older men who have had problems with their skin are acutely aware of the dangers, but younger men tend to view themselves as invincible and ignore warnings. Unless their employers have protection policies, young men often don't wear shirts or hats when working outside. And, according to the AAD and CDC (1996), they are less likely to wear sunscreens than older men, or if they do, they are less likely to use a product with SPF 15 or greater.

In outdoor jobs like construction, other risks are given priority. Accidental death and injury is a greater and more immediate concern. There are 13.3 accidental job-related deaths per 100,000 full-time workers in the United States. The dangers of skin cancer are neglected (Conlan 2003).

Outdoor Workers Receive Little Information on Sun Protection

Again, it is relevant that when looking at one of the biggest outdoor industries, most workers are men. Our belief is that education about sun protection and skin cancer prevention and detection should be targeted to all outdoor workers, but particularly men. Otherwise, there is a strong possibility that warnings will be ignored. Halpern and Kopp (2004) conducted a study in seven different countries and found that outdoor workers reported the lowest use of sunscreen of all respondents. This study included Australia, where sun protection education is highest, and still men in outdoor jobs ignore the message. Why is this?

Without delving into psychology, we believe there are many factors. In the United States, where education about sun safety is still lacking, the golden, muscled body image continues to be paramount. Further, most men are not taught to think about and care for their bodies the way women are. It is "sissy" to worry about a scar from a scrape or to care about what a mole looks like. The rough-and-tough look of weathered skin shows you are manly. To be pale is to be a weakling. Cultural stereotypes and lessons learned in childhood are hard to change. Many men do nothing to prevent sun damage, and

More than a million Americans develop skin cancer each year (AAD 2004c).

few notice changes to their skin. Those who do notice changes may choose to ignore them, believing they are insignificant.

Prevailing Attitudes Discourage Sun Protection

The International Life Saving Federation issued a statement that all professional and volunteer lifeguard organizations should have comprehensive, mandatory sun protection policies (ILSF 2004). The response from lifeguards, most of whom were between eighteen and twenty-five, was reported at a sun conference in California. Most of those who responded felt that the issues of sun protection and safety had been well presented to all lifeguards, that there was plenty of ongoing information given to them, and that sun safety was well presented to the public. But still, more than 50 percent of the lifeguards were content to be "sun worshippers" and didn't think they should be required to follow any particular method of sun protection (Brewster 1997).

Men Have Misperceptions about Using Sun Protection

A survey of outdoor workers by Wooley, Buettner, and Lowe (2002) found that many men assumed sun protective clothing, such as hats or loose-fitting shirts with long sleeves, is hot. In fact, the opposite is true: being covered by loose-fitting clothing when exposed to the sun is ultimately cooler. You need only to look at the clothing worn in some of the hottest countries in the world—Egypt, Singapore, and India—to realize the truth in this.

Another misperception found by the same survey was that if sunscreen is applied in the morning, it provides protection all day. We'll discuss this more completely in chapter 11, but we want to emphasize here that sunscreen must be reapplied every two hours during outdoor exposure. Further, some of the men surveyed didn't apply the sunscreen fifteen to twenty minutes before being exposed,

We estimate that approximately 10,250 Americans
will die from skin cancer in 2005.

or they said they simply don't put sunscreen on at all. Others said they avoid using it because it is too greasy.

Conlan (2003) makes note of a case of a seventy-four-year-old man who had spent his career as a construction surveyor in a high desert area under a blistering sun. In one year alone, he had ninety-three skin cancers taken off his forehead, arms, neck, and the backs of his hands.

Education about sun protection is essential for outdoor workers. Skin cancer detection and the importance of early treatment should be part of that education.

How Outdoor Workers Can Protect Themselves

Skin cancer has become an increasingly common problem among outdoor workers, and more and more employers are taking action to provide sun protection. For example, the California Department of Fish and Game regularly incorporates information about the use of sunscreen, protective clothing, and proper head attire into staff communications and safety newsletters. Education about skin cancer prevention and detection is being introduced at other organizations through labor organizations, employers, and employee groups. Policies are being initiated at state and federal levels, and adherence is becoming better enforced. However, as is true of education in the schools, all these efforts need media exposure and campaign efforts at local, state, and national levels to be most effective over the long term.

It is ultimately up to the individual to use as much sun protection as possible during a workday outside. Large employers may be aware of sun safety issues but slow to respond, while small employers may not yet even be aware of the issues. If you work outdoors, you should know how to protect yourself, and you should make it a point to talk to your employer about sun safety.

One cup of milk contains about 25 percent of the daily requirement for vitamin D.

The acronym AWARE is easy to remember and can be applied to methods of protection for outdoor workers.

A—avoid unprotected exposure at any time and especially during peak UVR hours

W—wear a long-sleeve shirt, a hat with a wide brim, and sunglasses; seek shade whenever possible

A—apply sunscreen with an SPF of 30 or higher, and reapply it every two hours as long as you are outdoors

R—routinely check your skin for changes

E—express the need for sun protection to your employer and your coworkers

. . . .

How Employers Can Help Protect Workers

Different labor organizations have been addressing the problem of workers being exposed to UVR for many years. The Occupational Safety and Health Administration (OSHA) of the U.S. Department of Labor wrote an interpretation to their Personal Protective Equipment standard in 1992. They stated that employers have a duty to protect workers from harmful exposure. While the standard does not require employers to supply sunscreen, it does specify that employees must wear sun protective clothing such as long-sleeve shirts and wide-brimmed hats (Conlan 2003). Other labor and union organizations have been making similar amendments. We believe responsible employers will do everything possible to protect workers from unprotected exposure to UVR, including supplying sunscreen with a minimum SPF of 15—ideally 30—and encouraging workers to use it and reapply it every two hours while outdoors.

Ten to twenty percent of actinic keratoses develop into squamous cell carcinomas (Odom 2004).

Work with Employees to Develop Sun Protection Strategies

Every outdoor job has different challenges for sun safety. To meet these challenges, employers should work with employees or employee representatives to develop policies and strategies that are tailored to specific jobs—including employees in the discussion of sun safety raises awareness throughout the organization. You may discover protection issues that you were unaware of. Look closely at each work area with your employees, taking into account reflected UVR, average daily UVR ratings, and shade. Work together to find the best sun protection for all workers. The following are some specific suggestions:

* Clear glass has an SPF of only 10 to 15 and does not block UVA. An employee sitting in the cabin of a crane is getting burned. Tinted glass could be installed and long sleeves worn with sunscreen on the face and the backs of the hands. Sunglasses should also be worn.

* Sun sleeves, which typically fit over the left arm of the driver or equipment operator, can also provide protection.

* Sunscreen gallon pump dispensers are available, as are sunscreen towelettes. These can be kept in locker areas, vehicle cabs, bathrooms, and other common areas. The more accessible the sunscreen, the more often it will be used.

* Safety helmets are available with a front peak and a legionnaire flap that covers the ears and neck.

* Company-issued sunglasses are another proven method of sun safety.

Actinic keratoses are more common in men under fifty (Odom 2004).

Incorporate Suggestions into a Well-Thought-Out Strategy

Once employers are aware of the problems associated with UVR exposure, they will want to develop strategies to help protect workers. First and foremost, employers can establish an education program for outdoor workers. Sun protective clothing, hats, and sunscreen should be provided, and workers should be encouraged to use them. Employers can initiate an incentive program to promote good sun safety habits, ensuring that adequate rewards are available for the program.

Other practical suggestions include relocating outdoor work to a shady area, changing schedules to avoid exposure between 10:00 A.M. and 4:00 P.M., providing indoor workspace, or using canopies, tents, or other portable structures to provide temporary shade.

Company leadership or management must take responsibility for the overall program, including education, availability of resources, monitoring of compliance, and group tactics. Employers should conduct a regular formal evaluation of the program, including written plans for improvement each year.

Employers should consider offering on-site skin cancer screenings.

Workplace Sun Protection Programs

Several organizations have initiated programs for sun protection education and skin cancer detection in the workplace. We have listed a few below, each with a short, general description. You can request more information directly from each organization (see "Online Resources").

Sun sense: skin cancer control for laborers. This program was developed by the Laborers' Health and Safety Fund of North America. It is a cancer awareness program focusing on incidence, causes, and risk factors as well as detection, prevention, and treatment.

There are many alternatives to tanning, such as airbrush tanning or self-tanners.

The pocket card. OSHA provides a pocket card of sun safety suggestions. The card gives generic information that can be used by all outdoor workers. It explains the best methods of protection, lists risk factors, and provides links for other sources of information.

The sun safety kit. The Skin Cancer Prevention Unit of the California Department of Health Services (CDHS) put together a comprehensive sun safety kit that can be used anywhere in the country as a model for educating outdoor workers. The kit includes publications produced by The Skin Cancer Foundation and information from the AAD in addition to the materials developed by the CDHS. It also includes posters showing outdoor workers protecting themselves from the sun, charts giving UVR levels, sunscreen samples, and a video.

Solar safe. This program was developed for the National Aeronautics and Space Administration workforce. It provides a comprehensive example of how sun protection education and skin cancer prevention and detection can be introduced into the workplace.

When Skin Cancer Is a Work-Related Injury

While it is one of the more difficult links to prove, more and more cases are being brought seeking compensation for work-related development of skin cancers. The arguments against compensation are that sun exposure in childhood leads to skin cancer later in life and that individuals spend significant leisure time in the sun. However, more employers are being held accountable for having sun protection policies that ensure their work environment in no material way contributes to diseases such as melanoma. Claims have been upheld and benefits awarded over the past decade in the United States because some level of causal relationship was established between a worker's employment and the development of skin cancer. For example, workers' compensation boards or state supreme courts have made awards to employees in New York, Texas, and Pennsylvania.

Airbrush tanning and self-tanners work best if you exfoliate your skin before use.

California has gone even further. California Labor Code 3212.11 now states that "skin cancer developing and manifesting itself (in publicly employed lifeguards) shall be presumed to arise out of and in the course of employment." So, for lifeguards in California, the onus is now on the employer to prove that skin cancer did not arise from the workplace.

The numbers of these cases will no doubt increase around the country with the increase in diagnosed cases of skin cancer, particularly melanoma. Employers should be AWARE of the problems associated with sun exposure and act responsibly to help prevent them.

Summing Up

Outdoor workers, particularly men, should be AWARE that they are at high risk for skin cancer and should be targeted for education about sun protection and skin cancer detection. Men are diagnosed with melanoma more often than women, and outdoor workers more often than any other segment of the population. Employers should commit to provide a sun safe environment, and all outdoor workers should learn and practice sun protection methods.

Our own survey of dermatologists at the 2004 meeting of the American Academy of Dermatology revealed that 34 percent would ban tanning beds.

baby boomers need sun protection and education

If you are a baby boomer or an older adult, you may have already experienced some form of skin cancer or know someone who has. Adults over the age of fifty have the greatest risk of developing skin cancers, particularly melanoma (Jemal et al. 2001). If you have had skin cancer, then your doctor has probably explained the importance of consistent sun protection and you are AWARE of the different methods to use.

If you are lucky enough not to have had skin cancer or other sun-related skin problems, but you know of the potential dangers, you may be thinking, *What's the point? I've already fried my skin, so why worry about it now?* It is never too late to protect your skin, and by doing so, you may potentially reverse some of the damage.

Think of it this way. Over the years, you may have harmed your skin's ability to repair cell damage, and cells may be more vulnerable. Therefore, now is the time you should be even more careful to use sun protection and to give yourself routine body checks. If you take care of your skin now, some of your skin's resiliency may return and further damage will be averted.

Baby boomers and older adults need immediate education about sun exposure. This age group is the most likely to be diagnosed with skin cancer, yet many are still unaware that it is a threat. Compounding the problem is the fact that this age group is the toughest to reach without the help of the media.

A national media campaign about skin cancers—including ads specifically targeted to baby boomers and older adults—could boost the use of prevention methods and could help lower mortality rates by providing information about detection.

. . . .

Four Easy Rules for Baby Boomers

Until such a campaign is developed, you should

* watch for any suspicious changes to your skin,

* accept that damage has been done but can be partially reversed,

* use sun protection to avoid adding to potential problems, and

* educate your children and grandchildren.

Rule 1: Watch for Changes

This may be the most important rule for baby boomers. In Australia, many baby boomers' lives have been saved because they were educated to catch changes early.

After the age of forty, skin seems to change fairly quickly, especially if your youth was spent in the sun. Many of the changes are normal and associated with age, while others are not. At this stage in life, if you have not already done so, you should establish a routine of monthly self-examinations and annual visits to the dermatologist or

Forty-two percent of dermatologists would prefer to have the tanning salon industry subject to mandatory federal regulation.

to a skin cancer screening. Middle-aged and older men should be encouraged to check themselves and have someone else check them, because they are least likely to detect melanoma in its early stages, when it is almost always curable through surgical removal.

We presented the steps for performing a monthly self-exam in chapter 6. Keep your records current and always remember the ABCDs of melanoma (asymmetry, border, color, and diameter). If a mole has changed or you have changes in your skin that seem abnormal, do not delay seeking treatment.

Skin Cancer Screenings

Since 1985, the AAD has coupled education about melanoma and skin cancer with free skin cancer screening programs throughout the United States. Volunteer dermatologists perform skin examinations, make recommendations, and give educational material to anyone who participates.

Studies have found that these free screenings are especially helpful for older men. During the first fifteen years of AAD screenings, from 1985 to 2000, 44 percent of the screened individuals diagnosed with melanoma were men over age fifty, though this group accounted for only 25 percent of those screened (Geller et al. 2003). Most of the melanomas found were not invasive, but without the screening, they might have remained undetected until dangerously advanced.

Women in this age group tend to find skin abnormalities quickly but may delay having them checked by a doctor, often because they do not have a regular dermatologist. Again, the skin cancer screening program offered by the AAD is an effective alternative.

Skin cancer screenings are generally held during the month of May and continue through the summer months, although in many states they are held periodically throughout the year. "Melanoma Monday," the first Monday in May, is a recently established awareness program that is used to alert the media of upcoming screenings. The screenings are promoted nationally and locally through posters, newspaper advertisements, and public service announcements on radio and television. Specific location information is provided by the AAD and The Skin Cancer Foundation. These screenings are sporadic, so if you discover a suspicious mole or

Tanning beds use UVA, which may cause harm at a deeper level than UVB.

change to your skin, do not wait for a screening to have it checked by a physician. See "Online Resources" for more information.

Rule 2: Accept That Damage Has Been Done

You may look at yourself in the mirror and wonder what all the hoopla is about. You've got a few wrinkles and a few patches of uneven pigmentation, but you use moisturizers and think your skin looks fine. If you are a woman, you may find that foundation evens out tone and skin color, and you don't really care too much about the wrinkles. If you are a man, you may think you look just a little more rugged. But you don't see any "real" damage, you simply see yourself getting older.

Don't believe your eyes. The damage may be there even if you can't see it. Fair-skinned baby boomers are unlikely to have known about sun protection or the risks of sun exposure during their early years. In fact, most baby boomers had lots of exposure through tanning. Baby boomers of color are also unlikely to have protected themselves. African-Americans, Latinos, and Asians in this age group are less likely to develop melanoma than whites, but statistics are showing a rise in skin cancer among all groups (SEER 2001). Further, people of color tend to fare worse with the disease because it is generally detected at later stages.

To convince yourself that the damage is there and the risk is high, ask your dermatologist to use an *ultraviolet color camera,* which instantly shows skin conditions including sun damage, skin infections, dead skin, dry skin, and excess oil. The amount of sun damage this camera reveals will alert your dermatologist to your risk for skin cancer and will probably motivate you to use sun protection methods.

Rule 3: Use Sun Protection to Avoid Adding to Potential Problems

Fair-skinned baby boomers who spent a lot of time unprotected in the sun should probably accept the fact that skin cells are damaged

UVA radiation is suspected to have links to melanoma and immune system damage.

or weakened and that further exposure could prompt the cells to mutate and become cancerous. Further, research suggests that having several sunburns over the course of a lifetime can double or triple the melanoma risk, no matter when the sunburn occurs (Pfahlberg, Kolmel, and Gefeller 2001). So a sunburn during middle age or later may be the one that triggers the cancer. It is equally important to understand that when they are protected from further exposure, weakened cells may still form skin cancers but at least they won't be "encouraged." And, ultimately, protection may help partially reverse some of the damage.

Women May Have Temporary Protection

Women between the ages of forty-five and sixty have much lower rates of diagnosed melanoma than men. This is interesting, because melanoma is more common than any non-skin-related cancer among women twenty-five to twenty-nine and second only to breast cancer for women thirty to thirty-four. Researchers at the University of California Irvine College of Medicine believe that hormonal changes due to menopause are the main reason that the risk decreases during these years (Beddingfield et al. 2002). This does not mean that further sun damage occurring during this period won't trigger skin cancers in later years; it simply means the risk of developing melanoma is lower during menopausal years.

Baby Boomer Men Must Be Especially Vigilant

Men between the ages of forty-five and sixty are significantly more likely than women to be diagnosed with melanoma (SCF 2003b). Whether this is because they lack the hormonal protection, or because they continue unprotected exposure, or because they had more exposure during their youth can't be determined. It is safe to say, however, that protection at this age is crucial.

Men in this age group have the poorest track record for performing monthly skin self-examinations or regularly visiting a dermatologist (Geller et al. 2003). Baby boomers and older adults must be AWARE of all sun protection methods and use them consistently.

Being tan is a sign that you are unhealthy rather than healthy.

Rule 4: Educate Your Children and Grandchildren

To date, most sun protective clothing in the United States is sold to people over forty-five. The buyers are generally people who have already experienced some form of skin cancer or other sun-related skin problem. They have learned that further exposure can trigger more problems and that the best protection is to cover up. Many of these people have received their education the hard way.

Conversely, most sun protective clothing in Australia is purchased by parents for their children. Prevention is a key concern of the national anti–skin cancer campaigns in Australia. The young and the aging are the two main targets, while everyone gets the message. We would like to see a similar campaign in this country, but until then, members of the baby boom generation can help lead the way by educating their own families.

We believe the best education comes from family. Stop by your dermatologist's office and get the literature about skin cancer prevention and detection. Find sun protective clothing on the Internet and give it to your children and grandchildren for birthdays and holidays. (We'll discuss protective clothing in more detail in chapter 12; see "Online Resources" for retailers.) Make sure your children understand that the only prevention is protection, and reinforce that message by telling your own story.

Summing Up

Baby boomers are at the highest risk of all age groups for developing skin cancers. Education about detection is crucial. Being AWARE and following good sun protection practices may help prevent additional problems.

More than a million people visit a tanning booth every day in America (Sekula-Gibbs 2004).

✳ PART III ✳

protecting yourself

✳ 11 ✳

using sunscreen effectively

The evolution of sunscreens has been full of promise and contradiction. Around the world, there are thousands of different brands of sunscreens with billions of dollars of research and development behind them. People who are concerned about protecting their skin use sunscreens, although many don't fully understand them. What is SPF? How much sunscreen should be used? Are lotions for children different than lotions for adults? Can sunscreen be used in the water? Does it work all day? Is sunscreen still important if the skin is already tan? The list of questions goes on and on. In addition, most people fail to use sunscreen properly and as a result are not effectively protected against the sun.

In this chapter, we clarify common misunderstandings and give advice about how to use sunscreens most effectively. We are greatly concerned that too many people rely solely on sunscreen for protection and then fail to use it correctly. We hope this chapter will show you how to use sunscreen properly and convince you that even when used correctly, sunscreen is only part of the solution.

. . . .

Confusion About Sunscreen Has Compromised Its Effectiveness

Between the 1950s and 1970s, research around the world firmly established the relationship between UVR exposure and skin cancers. The public began hearing more about the need to protect skin from burning, and pharmaceutical firms developed many new products promising protection.

In the early 1970s, the SPF system was introduced in the United States by the FDA. SPF indicates the amount of protection a sunscreen offers, but the public misunderstood it to be a method to calculate how many more hours you could be in the sun without burning. With SPF as high as 50, people assumed one application would last all day. Few paid attention to the directions to reapply every two hours.

By the 1990s, advertising had made people increasingly aware of the need to use sun protection—especially for children—but the whole topic of sunscreen was confusing. The AAD worked tirelessly to get clarification for the public, but when the FDA, dermatologists, and the sunscreen companies argued about how high the SPF rating could go, the public scratched its collective head and just figured the higher, the better. Some sunscreens were lotions, some gels, some sprays. You could only guess which one would work best.

Sunscreens had been developed based on a scientific belief that only the burn from UVB was harmful. Tanning salons began advertising that UVB was bad but UVA was fine—an argument they continue to put forward today. There was some mention of skin cancers, but most people believed that by using sunscreen, they were keeping their skin young and healthy.

By 2000 some scientists made the argument that sunscreen use was actually having the unintended effect of *increasing* skin cancer rates. How could it? Had people been given false information? What went wrong? The remainder of this chapter addresses some of the many questions and misperceptions consumers have about sunscreens today.

In 2004, 2,340 people in the United States died of nonmelanoma skin cancers (AAD 2004c).

. . . .

What Is Sunscreen?

Sunscreens are over-the-counter pharmaceutical products specifically designed for sun protection. They are regulated by the FDA, but no prescription is needed. They are effective when used with other sun protection methods but should never be used as the sole method of protection.

There are currently sixteen active ingredients approved by the FDA for use in sunscreens in the United States. (Avobenzone, approved in 1996, was the most recent addition to the list.) These active ingredients fall into two broad categories. Most are chemical absorbers for either UVB or UVA. A few are reflectors, sometimes also called "blockers."

Absorbers create a chemical reaction within the skin that allows the sunscreen to absorb the UVR before it reaches the skin. Octyl methoxycinnamate (OMC), homosalate, and octocrylene absorb UVB, and oxybenzone and avobenzone absorb UVA. *Reflectors* are physical barriers to the UV rays and block or reflect them away from the skin. These sunscreens usually contain zinc oxide or titanium dioxide. Today, many sunscreens contain a mixture of absorbers and reflectors.

In recent years, many sunscreens have been offered with new base formulations and new methods of application. Sunscreens are available in creams, mousses, lotions, and moisturizers. Hypoallergenic and waterproof products are also available.

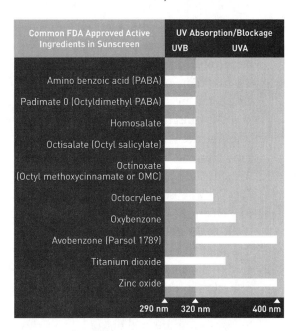

figure 11.1: Common Sunblock Ingredients

In Australia, car commercials advertise the UVR protection of windshields.

. . . .

Understanding SPF

SPF, or sun protection factor, is meant to measure the protection provided by a sunscreen. It is defined as the ratio of how long it takes for skin to redden with sunscreen compared to without sunscreen. For example, with an SPF 15 sunscreen, it will take your skin fifteen times longer to redden than it would without the sunscreen, assuming the same UVR exposure. So if your skin would redden in five minutes without sunscreen, then it will redden after seventy-five minutes with an SPF 15 sunscreen. It's easy to see why most people interpreted SPF as telling them how much longer they could stay in the sun. But that is not how you should interpret it.

SPF Indicates Percentage of UVR Blocked

Here's an alternate way to understand SPF. An SPF 15 sunscreen, when it is applied properly, will absorb or block fourteen out of fifteen units of UVR. It doesn't absorb the fifteenth unit. This is why when you use an SPF 15 sunscreen, it will take fifteen times as long for your skin to redden as without the sunscreen. Similarly, an SPF 30 sunscreen absorbs twenty-nine out of thirty units of UVR. The thirtieth unit is not absorbed, so when you use an SPF 30 sunscreen, it takes thirty times as long for your skin to redden as without the sunscreen.

Now, absorbing fourteen out of fifteen units of UVR is absorbing 93 percent of UVR, and absorbing twenty-nine out of thirty units of UVR is absorbing 97 percent of UVR. So an SPF 15 sunscreen, when it is applied properly, protects you against 93 percent of UVR, while an SPF 30 sunscreen protects you against 97 percent of UVR. And an SPF 50 sunscreen will protect you against 98 percent of UVR. So when you move from SPF 15 to SPF 30, you aren't doubling your protection—you are making only a modest improvement, from 93 percent protection to 97 percent protection. And going from SPF 30 to SPF 50 is only going from 97 percent protection to 98 percent

Within ten years, melanoma may be diagnosed more often than lung cancer in the Sun Belt.

protection. That's a more realistic way to compare the protection you get from different SPF-rated sunscreens.

SPF Only Indicates UVB Protection

There are some other important issues to understand about SPF. The next issue is that the SPF rating only tells you about protection from UVB. The reason is that the reddening of your skin (erythemal response) used to rate the SPF of a sunscreen is caused by UVB. UVB is present primarily from 10:00 A.M. to 4:00 P.M., it is greatest in the summer or in places closer to the equator, and it does not travel through glass. Your skin responds to UVB exposure with a delayed burn three to four hours later. However, scientists now believe UVA causes many other skin problems that don't show up as quickly. UVA is present in nearly the same levels year-round and all day long. It can pass more readily through clouds and glass. The problems caused by UVA can take many years to become apparent, but they are quite real and quite serious. So, in order to get protection against both UVA and UVB, you should select a sunscreen that says it provides multispectrum protection, broad-spectrum protection, or UVA/UVB protection—not just a sunscreen with a high SPF (UVB) rating.

Reapply Sunscreen Every Two Hours Regardless of SPF

There are two other common mistakes people make in interpreting SPF ratings. First, sunscreen must be reapplied every two hours regardless of SPF level. Don't go longer between applications with an SPF 50 than you would with an SPF 15. Whether the sunscreen is an SPF 15 or SPF 30 or SPF 50, it has to be reapplied every two hours while exposed to the sun to maintain its protection level. The reason is that exposure to UVR is actually degrading the active ingredients in the sunscreen, and any sunscreen—regardless of rating—will have lost much of its effectiveness after two hours of UVR exposure. Only the physical blockers, such as zinc oxide, maintain high levels of

Ancient humans understood the need to protect themselves from the sun.

protection for more than two hours, and very few sunscreens rely solely on physical blockers. So reapply your sunscreen every two hours.

High-SPF Sunscreen Does Not Make Prolonged Exposure Safe

Second, don't stay in the sun for a long time because you are using a high-SPF sunscreen. A high-SPF sunscreen is really giving only a modest increase in protection over a lower-SPF sunscreen, and you can't always be sure you have applied it sufficiently to all exposed skin or that you have reapplied it as often as you should. Prolonged exposure increases the risk of skin cancers, including melanoma. Use sunscreen, but avoid staying in the sun for extended periods of time.

. . . .
How to Use Sunscreen Properly

This issue is so important we have devoted an entire section to it. A lack of understanding of when, how often, and how much sunscreen should be applied is the primary reason many scientists and doctors say sunscreens don't work in practice or don't work as well as advertised.

Firstly, sunscreen should be applied twenty minutes before you go outside. This allows time for it to penetrate or bind to the skin.

Secondly, you need to use an adequate amount of sunscreen in order for it to be effective. It is estimated that most people underapply sunscreen by as much as 50 percent of the recommended amount (AAD 1999a). Therefore, a sunscreen with an SPF label of 15 may in practice be providing an SPF of only 7 or 8. If you underapply sunscreen and stay in the sun too long, you will likely get sunburned—which appears to be exactly what most people do. Almost 75 percent of people who use sunscreen end up sunburned because they fail to use the sunscreen properly (Wright, Wright, and Wagner 2001).

To achieve effective sun protection, an adult should use approximately one ounce of sunscreen to cover the entire body every two

UVR, visible light, and infrared rays are all part of
the electromagnetic radiation spectrum.

hours. Cover all exposed areas liberally. Pay special attention to ears, nose, feet, hands, bald spots, back of neck, arms, and legs. A typical tube containing three to five ounces of sunscreen might be enough for only one day at the beach for one person.

A family of four (two adults and two children) spending six hours a day on the beach (three applications of sunscreen per person) for six days should use at least two four-ounce bottles of sunscreen per day, or twelve bottles during the six days. This can be cut down substantially by wearing sun protective clothing and using sunscreen only on exposed skin. Remember that lips can burn, and use a lip balm sunscreen of SPF 15 or higher.

Thirdly, even if a label promises "all-day protection," sunscreen should be reapplied every two hours until sunset. It should be reapplied after swimming or sweating, and it should be reapplied if it has been rubbed off. Reapplying sunscreen does not increase the SPF—it just keeps the SPF at its maximum level.

Fourthly, always check the label for an expiration date. Sunscreen ingredients lose their effectiveness over time, and expired sunscreen must be replaced. Do not use sunscreen that was left over from last summer. Throw it away and get a new bottle. Then start using it every day, even in winter.

Which Sunscreens Offer the Best Protection?

Broad-spectrum sunscreens that block both UVA and UVB may be more effective in preventing squamous cell cancers and its precursors than those that block only UVB. Used with other sun protection methods, broad-spectrum sunscreen may also help reduce the risk of melanoma.

Select an appropriate sunscreen SPF based on your skin type and how long you anticipate being in the sun. In general, a sunscreen with SPF 30 or higher that is also labeled "broad-spectrum" or "UVA and UVB"—used with sun protection clothing, hats, and sunglasses—will give the maximum protection available when you are outdoors.

X-rays are the form of electromagnetic radiation
with the shortest wavelength.

Another commonsense element in selecting the best sunscreen is to make sure you are comfortable with how the sunscreen feels on your skin so that you are more likely to use it. Try different products until you find a sunscreen that feels good to you and that you want to use regularly.

Nearly all sunscreens rely on a combination of active ingredients. As the scientific understanding of UVR, the skin, and sunscreen has advanced, the combinations of active ingredients in sunscreens have changed. For example, sunscreens that used to be called "sunblocks" but are now more often labeled "full-spectrum sunscreens" typically contained zinc oxide. These products were broad-spectrum, extremely safe, and effective, but using them was like applying white paint, and so they lost popularity. However, newer products contain microfine particles of zinc that are almost invisible on the skin. These newer formulations have gained in popularity and are now recommended by many dermatologists because they help to minimize the harmful effects of UVB and UVA on DNA and on important proteins such as collagen, elastin, and keratin, which keep skin smooth and firm.

Water-resistant sunscreens are recommended for many sports. They have a high concentration of lipid-soluble UVR-absorbing chemicals that adhere well to the skin and are not easily washed off by sweat or water.

People of all colors should use a sunscreen with an SPF of at least 15. SPF lower than 15 does not prevent tanning and therefore does not offer protection against damage to DNA. This is true for all skin types. People with skin types I, II, and III should use a broad-spectrum sunscreen with an SPF of 30 or higher.

. . . .

Should Children Use Sunscreens?

Children can and should use sunscreens as soon as they turn six months. Regular use of sunscreen throughout childhood reduces the total amount of UVR absorbed by the skin, which in turn will help prevent premature aging of the skin and reduces the risk of all skin

Ultraviolet radiation is electromagnetic radiation with a wavelength shorter than visible light but longer than X-rays.

cancers. The American Academy of Pediatrics approves the use of sunscreen on infants younger than six months when adequate clothing and shade is not available (AAPCEH 1999).

Sunscreen should always be used with other protection methods. When they are outside, children should wear sun protective clothing, including a hat with a three-inch brim; sunglasses; and sunscreen on any exposed parts of the body.

There are many different types of sunscreens that have been made to be appealing to children. Those with zinc and titanium dioxide are frequently recommended and come in different colors and dispensers to make them more "fun." Children should also wear lip balm of at least SPF 15.

Sunscreen for children presents some difficulties:

* Sunscreens must be reapplied every two hours while exposed to UVR to be effective. School or day care policies may not allow this.

* Parents and caregivers often misunderstand SPF and allow children to stay outside too long.

* It is difficult to get children to allow you to put the sunscreen on. They often rub it off or squirm so much it is unevenly applied.

* Parents and caregivers often think sunscreen is the only protection children need.

* Parents are responsible for checking policies about sunscreen at schools or day care.

Given these problems, many pediatricians have been concerned that sunscreens are used incorrectly and that it may encourage parents to allow their children to be outside longer than they should be. The AAP now recommends that "the first and best line of defense against the sun is covering up" (2004). Hats, sunglasses, and clothing are suggested as the primary methods of protection, followed by the use of shade and sunscreen.

Sun protective clothing usually blocks 97 percent of UVR.

If you think of sunscreen as a lifesaving medication for your children, you will be more likely to use it properly. Teach your children to avoid unprotected exposure at all times but particularly between 10:00 A.M. and 4:00 P.M. Buy sun protective clothing and teach them the value of using it. Buy hats and sunglasses, allowing them to make their own choices from among sun protective styles. Use broad-spectrum SPF 30 sunscreen on all exposed skin, even on cloudy days. Reapply sunscreen every two hours while exposed, and teach them to reapply while exposed even on cloudy days.

Is Sunscreen Needed Year-Round?

Many dermatologists recommend using sunscreen every day throughout the year, regardless of your skin color. Moreover, people with skin types I through IV living between zero degrees and forty-five degrees north or south latitude should absolutely use effective sunscreens daily year-round. While those with type V or VI skin might not have to wear sunscreens during the winter, they should be careful of reflected UVR from snow and ice (Pathak 2002). Sunscreen should be used on both sunny days and overcast days, because harmful UVR can pass through clouds and fog. The safest approach for people of all skin types is to use sunscreen on exposed skin all year.

Do Moisturizers and Makeup Containing Sunscreen Really Work?

Many moisturizers and makeup products have sunscreens in them that are effective. Most are SPF 15, but you can find some with SPF 30. Look for broad-spectrum. Makeup with sunscreen must be evenly spread to be effective. The best assurance is to put sunscreen on first, give it time to be absorbed, then apply makeup.

Infrared radiation is the form of electromagnetic radiation with the shortest wavelength.

The Misunderstanding or Misconception about Base Tans

Many believe that getting a "base tan" will prevent sunburn and protect against skin cancers. This misperception has been used by the tanning bed industry to attract customers. All tans are damage to skin. What is called "protection" provided by a base tan would equal an SPF of about 2, which is so low it is counterproductive (Pathak 1999). You may prevent burning, but you have increased your chances of getting skin cancer. Avoid getting tanned or burned.

Summing Up

Be AWARE that sunscreen is only one of several methods of sun protection. It should always be used in combination with other methods such as sun protective clothing, hats, and sunglasses. The best sunscreens are broad-spectrum (blocking both UVA and UVB) with an SPF of 30 or higher. These recommendations will likely be revised over time as more research and knowledge become available.

UVA and UVB radiation penetrate the atmosphere, but UVC radiation does not.

sun protective clothing

While sun protective clothing is a relatively new concept in this country, in Australia it now sells almost three times as well as sunscreen. What is sun protective clothing? Why are many American pediatricians and dermatologists saying that it is better than sunscreen for protecting against UVR? Why do consumers like it? And where can you find it?

Common sense suggests that a physical block—clothing—is the best way to protect the skin from the sun. In chapter 2, we discussed the direct correlation between the change in clothing styles and the increase in skin cancers. The fewer clothes people wear, the more skin cancers they get.

. . . .
Why Do People Wear Sun Protective Clothing?

There are several practical reasons for choosing to use sun protective clothing:

Protection is reliable. Sun protective clothing protects you both consistently and constantly. Unlike sunscreen, the protection offered by UPF-rated clothing does not fade or wear off during the day.

Protection is less expensive. Clothing is bought only once and will last many seasons or until outgrown. Over the long term, buying sun protective clothing is less expensive than buying sunscreen.

Protection is not messy. Unlike sunscreen, sun protective clothing is not sticky, oily, allergenic, or difficult to apply. Sun protective clothing reduces the amount of sunscreen needed on exposed areas, such as the face or hands. This is particularly appealing to parents of young children and to men.

Protection is provided for both UVA and UVB. Unlike sunscreens, which have SPF ratings based only on UVB, clothing is rated for its protection against both UVA and UVB.

· ·

The History of Sun Protective Clothing

During the 1980s, when the epidemic of skin cancer in Australia became a national concern, the Anti-Cancer Council of Victoria introduced the "Slip, Slop, Slap" recommendations (slip on a shirt, slop on sunscreen, slap on a hat). Researchers quickly realized that while the recommendations were correct, many people were wearing T-shirts for protection, not knowing that the average protection offered by a cotton T-shirt is less than SPF 10.

The Anti-Cancer Council of Victoria quickly got to work finding material that would effectively block out the sun. They borrowed the concept of the surfer's "rash shirt" (worn to protect against skin burns that result from lying on the surfboard) and began marketing the first sun protective swim shirts. The shirt was followed by "neck-to-knee" swimsuits, which look very similar to wet suits, and a new industry—sun protective clothing—was born in Australia.

Carcinogens are substances known to cause cancer.

. . . .

The Ultraviolet Protection Factor Rating System

Soon entrepreneurs were busy making their own sun protective clothing. However, there were no industry standards in place to guarantee that the materials being used were in fact sun protective. Again, the Australian government intervened as part of its continued commitment to slowing the epidemic of skin cancer. Starting in 1992, the Australian Radiation Laboratory, which later became ARPANSA (the Australian Radiation Protection and Nuclear Safety Agency, an agency similar to the EPA in this country), developed regulatory standards for any garment claiming to be sun protective. ARPANSA rated garments according to UPF or ultraviolet protection factor, a rating system similar to SPF. Almost 4 million garments are now tested each year by ARPANSA and given tags indicating their UPF rating.

In 1998, the American Association of Textile Chemists and Colorists (AATCC) adapted the Australian UPF standard for use in the United States. Later, the American Society for Testing and Materials (ASTM) developed standards for simulating a sun protective garment's life cycle and for labeling a garment claiming to be sun protective. We estimate that currently, in the United States, nearly 1 million garments are tested each year using the AATCC and ASTM standards.

UPF rates the amount of UVR—both UVA and UVB—that is blocked by a fabric. UPF is a similar concept to SPF. UPF is the ratio of how much UVR is measured at a detector with the protection of a fabric compared to without the protection of a fabric. The detector is a machine: either a spectrophotometer or a spectroradiometer. If a fabric is rated UPF 30, then it is absorbing or blocking 29 out of 30 units of UVR, or 97 percent of UVR. This is the same as the level of protection provided by an SPF 30 sunscreen that is used properly.

There are some differences between the UPF rating for clothing and the SPF rating for sunscreens. For example, UPF is determined using a machine in a laboratory, whereas SPF often involves testing on people. UPF rates both UVA and UVB protection, whereas SPF

A nanometer is one billionth of a meter.

rates only UVB protection. Perhaps the biggest difference is that in practice, wearing a UPF 30 garment will actually protect you against 97 percent of UVR, whereas most people who use an SPF 30 sunscreen don't use it properly and end up with much less protection. A final important difference is that UPF involves voluntary industry standards, whereas SPF is an FDA program.

Testing

Most of us tend to trust manufacturers' claims about products because we have relied on the Federal Trade Commission or the FDA to monitor these claims. While sunscreens are regulated by the FDA, sun protective clothing is not. As a consumer, you are essentially relying on the integrity of the manufacturers' statements about their clothing. To accurately determine whether a fabric is sun protective, a manufacturer must carefully test it on special laboratory equipment. No one can tell the level of UVR protection of a fabric just by looking at it, because UVR and visible light do not pass through a fabric in the same way.

A complete and comprehensive set of tests would involve an initial UVR transmittance test, followed by laundering the garment forty times, exposing it to one hundred fading units of simulated sunlight, and retesting it for UVR transmittance. Garment ratings should be based on the lowest finding of the initial test and the second test, although many manufacturers only conduct an initial test. Two relevant test standards have been developed for UPF rating:

* AATCC Test Method 183 is the standard that describes how to conduct a UVR transmittance test.

* ASTM D 6544 is the standard that describes the methods for laundering and exposing fabric to simulated sunlight. It is a rigorous evaluation of the fabric's life-cycle UVR protection.

A UVC ray is between 100 and 280 nanometers long.

Labeling

Once testing has been performed, manufacturers can label their garments based on the test results recorded. ASTM D 6603 describes how a garment may be labeled. Elements include a UPF value and a classification category (good, very good, or excellent).

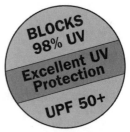

This garment fabric was independently tested using:

American Society for Testing and Materials D 6544 and American Association of Textile Chemists and Colorists Test Method 183 for the rigorous evaluation of a fabric's life cycle UV protection.

Australian/New Zealand Standard 4399 - the original, globally recognized standard for sun protective clothing.

This tag complies with American Society for Testing and Materials D 6603 for labeling sun protective clothing.

figure 12.1: Sample Label

Who Buys Sun Protective Clothing?

In Australia, the anti–skin cancer campaign was originally focused on prevention (by targeting children) and on early detection (by targeting seniors). Focusing on these two segments of the population was the fastest way to slow down the epidemic of skin cancers, including melanoma. As a result, the market for sun protective clothing was directed toward children in particular. Most children in Australia wear sun protective swimwear or beachwear. Most also wear protective sportswear and have sun protection garments included in school uniforms.

Interestingly, the American market appears the opposite. The main buyers of sun protective clothing in America are people forty or over—especially people who have experienced health problems from sun exposure, want to prevent a recurrence, and have received information from their doctors. The clothes are designed for everyday wear and adult activities. In addition, some parents are buying sun protective swimwear for their children.

This difference in buying patterns reflects the fact that there is no coordinated national skin cancer prevention campaign in America. Parents in the United States are still generally unaware of the

A UVB ray is between 280 and 315 nanometers long.

importance of consistent sun protection and the best methods to achieve it. When we see a change in the buying patterns—an equal amount of sun protective clothing bought for children and adults—we will know that parents are AWARE of the need for sun protection.

· ·

Shopping for Sun Protective Clothing

While the idea of wearing clothing for sun protection is not new, technology and design have pushed the idea to new levels. Fabrics and designs that have UPF ratings, provide excellent skin coverage, keep moisture away from the skin, and provide ventilation are becoming inexpensive and easily accessible. If the garment is sold as sun protective, read the labels carefully. Labels should include a UPF classification category (good, very good, or excellent), the UPF value (between 15 and 50+), and the statement "Product labeled according to ASTM D 6603." (See figure 12.1 for a sample label.) Standards in this industry are still voluntary, so you should always look for the test methods listed on the labels. Keep in mind that the tests only relate to the fabric—design, fit, and the amount of body covered are not considered when UPF ratings are given.

Evaluating Clothing That Is Not UPF Rated

Responding to the epidemic of skin cancers in Australia, the Anti-Cancer Council of Victoria (now Cancer Council Victoria) and the Australian Radiation Laboratory (now ARPANSA) conducted a joint survey in 1991 and found that not all clothing provided effective protection against UVR. Further research showed that many summer materials had protection factors as low as 5 to 10 (Gies et al. 1998). Very similar results were reported by a German team that tested 236 typical summer fabrics and also discovered that the majority of fabrics failed to protect as well as an SPF 30 sunscreen (Gambichler et al. 2001).

A UVA ray is between 315 and 400 nanometers long.

These fabrics have the same elements as American fabrics, which leads us to believe that similar testing in this country would have very similar results. When a garment isn't UPF rated, how can you know whether it will offer good UVR protection?

. . . .

Which Fabrics Are Sun Protective?

ARPANSA provides the following list of factors that can help you determine whether a garment will effectively block UVR.

Weave density. Less UVR passes through tightly woven or knitted fabrics. The smaller the spacing between the individual fiber strands, the higher the protection.

Color. Many dyes absorb UVR. Darker colors (black, navy, and dark red) of the same fabric type will usually absorb UVR more effectively than light pastel shades.

Tension. Stretching a fabric may decrease its effectiveness in blocking UVR. This is common in knitted or elasticized fabrics, and care should be taken to select the correct size for the wearer.

Moisture content. Many fabrics offer less UVR protection when wet. This is because UVR passes through water better than through air. The drop in protection when wet depends on the type of fabric and the amount of moisture it absorbs when wet.

Condition. Most fabrics will get less protective as they age, and old, threadbare, or faded garments will be less effective. The exception is that many brand-new cotton-based fabrics can actually offer more UVR protection after they have been washed at least once. Shrinkage in the fabric closes small gaps between the threads and allows less UVR to pass through.

Ozone depletion is the result of chlorofluorocarbons (CFCs).

Design

Whether or not the fabric is UPF rated, selecting garments that are sensibly designed for sun protection can make a large difference in your overall UVR exposure. Garments that provide more body coverage offer more protection. A shirt with long sleeves and a high collar offers more protection than a short-sleeve shirt without a collar. A legionnaire-style cap with a flap protects the ears and back of the neck much better than a baseball cap. A broad-brimmed hat shades the face and neck.

Comfort

When you consider the elements of fabric and design described above, it is easy to see how and why a fabric is sun protective. However, one essential element is missing from this list: comfort.

Tightly woven, dark, thick, heavy fabrics are hot. Sun protective clothing should be light, cool, and comfortable so that you will wear it and keep it on in hot conditions. Remember that the whole idea of sun protective clothing is to allow you to safely enjoy the outdoors. Look for clothing with wicking and ventilation properties.

Wicking. When clothing gets wet from perspiration, it sticks to the skin and hinders the evaporation process. Wicking or breathable fabric has special fibers and weaves to keep perspiration away from your skin.

Ventilation. This is an important feature of sun protective clothing. If the garment is well designed, it will have panels that allow for airflow. There is no single method for providing ventilation. However, always look for it in sun protective clothing that will be used for activewear.

Garment Types

Good sun protective clothing is carefully designed for comfort and maximum protection. Below, we describe some of the types of

CFCs were banned throughout the world in the 1970s.

sun protective garments that are available. Always consider the activity for which you will be wearing the garment, and that will help you determine the best design.

Surf shirts or rash shirts. These shirts offer superior sun protection to the upper body. They are usually made with a stretch nylon-Lycra or polyester fabric. They are designed to fit loosely to allow for evaporation, and they have high collars and long sleeves for coverage. The best are made from polyester so they are chlorine resistant and are rated to block 97 percent of UVR.

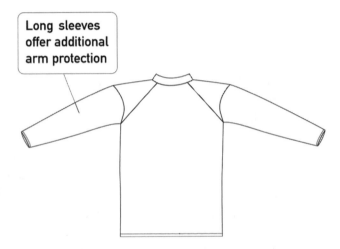

Long sleeves offer additional arm protection

figure 12.2: Surf Shirt

Neck to knee. These swimming garments look like wet suits with short legs and offer superior sun protection for arms, legs, and the trunk of the body. They are made to be worn in the water, usually with knitted nylon-Lycra or with polyester that is chlorine resistant. They should be rated to block 97 percent of UVR.

Athletic shirts. Most sun protection clothing companies will offer some type of athletic shirt. These shirts are meant to be worn while doing outdoor athletic activities such as jogging, hiking, or bike riding. Athletic shirts should be made with a lightweight wicking fabric and have plenty of ventilation.

The SPF system for rating sunscreens was established
in the United States in 1972.

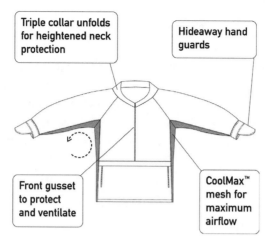

figure 12.3: Athletic Shirt

Everyday shirts and blouses. Beyond the sun protective fabrics, these garments usually have special features such as fold-up collars to protect the neck or roll-down cuffs to protect the hands. The best designs are stylish and lightweight with plenty of ventilation so they can be worn in the warmest climates.

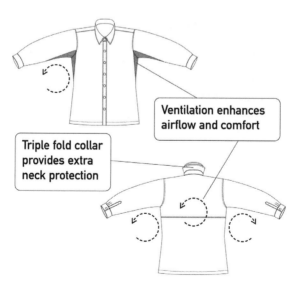

figure 12.4: Everyday Shirt

The tanning bed was invented in the 1970s.

Fabric Additives

In addition to garments specially designed for sun protection, there are additives that can be washed into ordinary garments to improve their UVR blockage. If you choose to try these additives, follow the directions carefully and repeat every few months. These additives generally work best for cottons and are not recommended for synthetics.

· ·

Where Can You Buy Sun Protective Clothing?

In "Online Resources," we have provided a list of retailers that sell sun protective clothing. Most offer Internet or catalog shopping. Most can be found online by using the search phrase "sun protective clothing." There are a few that have retail outlets. Check Web sites for locations.

Summing Up

Sun protective clothing provides the easiest and most effective method of sun protection. It is made for all ages and sizes and is highly recommended by dermatologists and other skin specialists. Be AWARE and use all sun protection methods together to help prevent skin cancers.

In the 1980s, fewer than 10,000 businesses ran tanning beds (Pouliot 2003).

a close look at hats

Conventional wisdom dictates that wearing a hat provides sun protection, and various studies support this wisdom. In Australia, a study at Queensland University showed the difference in the risk of getting skin cancer between people who wore a hat while farming and those who did not. Without the protection of a hat, the risk of getting nonmelanoma skin cancer was estimated to increase by up to one hundred times for basal cell carcinomas and thirteen times for squamous cell carcinomas (Wong, Airey, and Fleming 1996).

Another study in England measured the degree of sun protection provided by various styles of hats and found that a hat must have at least a three-inch brim to adequately protect the nose and cheeks (Diffey and Cheeseman 1992). Dermatologists and skin cancer organizations around the world concur with this finding. Today, recommendations for sun protective hats always state that the brim should be at least three inches wide. Only hats for infants are smaller.

Our focus in this chapter is to highlight the three most popular traditional hat styles, explain why they do not provide adequate sun protection, and provide suggestions for hats that offer the most effective sun protection. We'll discuss how to choose a hat for sun protection and show why a three-inch brim is essential. We'll provide information about current styles and materials for children's and adults' sun hats. Finally, we'll discuss school programs and legislation that are shaping policy for hats in schools.

. . . .

Traditional Hat Styles May Not Provide Sun Protection

As we mentioned in chapter 2, up until the second half of the twentieth century, most people in the United States tried to avoid sun exposure because tanned skin indicated outdoor labor or field work. Pale skin was a status symbol, especially for women. The bonnet, with its wide, downward-curving brim, offered complete sun protection for the entire face, and for about two hundred years, this was the most popular women's hat worn. While men wore hats that indicated both their profession and their social status, they were not so conscientious about keeping their skin pale. Unfortunately, as women cut their hair in accordance to the styles of the Roaring Twenties, the bonnet gave way to the cloche, which hugged the head like a helmet with a very small brim. And, as suntanning became a national pastime, hats declined in popularity.

Three types of hats are still commonly worn in the United States—straw hats, baseball caps, and ten-gallon hats—but unfortunately, none of these really provide adequate sun protection.

Straw Hats

A straw hat is probably the only casual hat for women that is still worn fairly regularly, usually at the beach or in the garden. The first American version was made in Providence, Rhode Island, when a fourteen-year-old girl copied an English straw bonnet she could not afford. She copied it so well that she received numerous commissions to make more, and the industry was born.

While straw hats are lightweight and comfortable, most do not provide adequate sun protection. The weave is usually too loose, allowing UVR to pass between the straw fibers. In addition, the straw reflects the UVR that bounces up from the ground back down onto the face. This is unfortunate because straw hats often have wide brims. For effective sun protection, straw hats must be tightly woven

By the year 2000, there were over 50,000 businesses running tanning beds (Pouliot 2003).

or lined with cloth. A cloth lining in a straw hat blocks direct UVR from above and absorbs indirect or reflected UVR from below.

Baseball Caps

From a fashion perspective, the baseball cap has truly survived the test of time. It became popular during the 1920s and 1930s, when fans began using their home-team baseball caps as everyday wear. Originally, the caps were shaped more like a skullcap, but baseball caps with visors gained widespread popularity when they were worn by Babe Ruth. The baseball cap is now an international symbol of America.

Many believe the baseball cap provides adequate sun protection for the face. Like the straw hat, it does not. Baseball caps protect only the top of the head, the forehead, and the top of the nose. They do not protect the back of the neck, the tops of the ears, the sides of the cheeks, or the chin. Even baseball caps with extended visors offer little protection to the sides of the cheeks or the chin, and they provide no protection to the back of the neck and the ears. Baseball caps should not be considered sun protective.

The Ten-Gallon Hat

The ten-gallon hat or Stetson, a Texas icon, was invented during the 1930s and has become well known throughout the world. John Batterson Stetson, who fought for the rights to market the hat from a company in England, added the *galons*—or braids—around the crown. Many misunderstood the word, and because the hat was so big, it became known as the "ten-gallon hat."

Usually made with heavy felt and leather, this hat is highly sun protective, but the shape of the hat and the way it is often worn may negate much of the protection. If worn properly, the ten-gallon hat protects the top of the head, the tops of the ears, the forehead, and the nose. However, when the sides are turned up, there is still exposure at the base of the ears and the lower cheeks. Further, many wear the hat tilted back, thus exposing much more skin.

Sun protective clothing should be part of uniforms for outdoor workers.

. . . .

Function vs. Fashion

Hats began making a comeback late in the twentieth century. We believe this was in direct response to the growing numbers of diagnosed skin cancers, not fashion direction. Hat sales statistics suggest that they are being worn primarily by middle-aged and elderly people—those most likely to have sun-related skin problems—and that the hats have wide brims and are more sun protective.

We also know that there is a growing movement to get children to wear hats. Schools are introducing them at recess, sporting programs are incorporating them into uniforms, and all anticancer education programs advocate their use.

Hats that are sun protective will no doubt become fashionable as more people become AWARE of the need to wear them.

. . . .

Choosing a Hat for Sun Protection

When you're choosing a hat for sun protection, you'll want to consider the width of the brim, the shape of the hat, and the material. Consider the activity for which you'll be wearing the hat, then choose a suitable style.

Why Hats Need a Three-Inch Brim to Be Protective

As we mentioned earlier, Wong, Airey, and Fleming (1996) conducted a study to determine how much UVR exposure could be reduced by wearing a hat. Their findings indicated that exposure to the forehead and to the nose was reduced significantly, but there was less reduction in exposure to the cheek.

These findings reveal that *without* a hat, the nose receives the highest annual exposure, or about 36 percent of the total ambient UVR. The study also highlights the fact that on a person who is

In the United Kingdom, parents are being sued under child abuse laws for allowing their children in tanning booths.

wearing a hat, the cheek is the area most exposed. The chin is another area that may receive high exposure even while a hat is worn.

Diffey and Cheeseman (1992) measured the extent of sun protection achieved by wearing different styles of hats. They tested a total of twenty-eight hats and found that

* all hats provide good protection to the forehead,

* hats with little or no brim provide poor protection at other sites on the head and neck, and

* a hat with at least a three-inch brim is necessary to provide reasonable protection around the nose and cheeks.

Hat Shapes and Reflected UVR

In addition to the size of a hat's brim, the shape of the brim is also very important. Hats with a three-inch or wider brim provide excellent protection against direct UVR (that is, UVR that travels in a straight line down from the sun to your head). However, UVR can also bounce back up off various surfaces. (We'll discuss reflected UVR more in chapter 15.) For example, on a sandy beach, there is significant reflected UVR. Hat shapes that protect better against reflected UVR are ones that curve down to follow the contours of your head and neck. For example, a legionnaire-style hat provides the best protection for your neck because the fabric flap lies on top of your skin and blocks both direct and reflected UVR.

As a general rule, the lower points on your face will be exposed to the most reflected UVR, while higher points will be exposed to less reflected UVR. For this reason, it is important to use sunscreen on your face—particularly on your chin and cheeks—even while wearing a hat with a three-inch brim. Without sunscreen, in situations where there are high levels of reflected UVR, even a hat with a five-inch brim will offer little protection to your chin.

Finally, some hats have dark underbrims. The dark color absorbs more of the reflected UVR and better protects your face.

France is the only country that bans children from using tanning booths.

Sun Protective Styles and Materials

You know that sun protective hats should have a three-inch brim, but how do you know what they should be made from? The material should be cool and durable. When you are buying a hat for sun protection, be sure to check the hangtag. The hat should be rated to block 97 percent UVR or more. This means that the manufacturer has sewn the hat together with material that has been tested or has lined the hat with tested material.

Hats should be comfortable. They should fit snugly but not too tightly, they should not be hot, and they should be good looking. The style of a hat can be both sun protective and attractive. Choose hats based on the activities they will be used for. Some are made with straw so they are lightweight, while others are made from cotton so they can be crushed in suitcases. There are a wide range of materials, styles, and uses. We have covered many in the following sections, and we hope you will always choose carefully in order to provide the best sun protection for you and your family.

. . . .

Hats for Children

Ideally, a good sun protective hat for children should shield as much of the face and neck as possible. Regardless of the style, the hat should be constructed of fabric that has a UPF of 30 or more, meaning that it blocks at least 97 percent of UVR.

Hats for Babies

Since young babies are usually lying down or reclining in car seats or strollers, their hats should be made from a soft fabric with a small brim. The baby's head is of particular concern when the child is riding in a baby backpack. Be sure to keep it covered. Because hats alone cannot provide complete protection, the tops of strollers should be tilted to provide maximum shade and you should always seek a shaded area for your baby when outside.

In 2004, one in thirty-seven Americans has a lifetime risk
of developing melanoma (AAD 2004c).

Hats for Toddlers and Young Children

Many parents complain that toddlers won't keep their hats on. If your children wear hats every time they go outside, it becomes a habit. Don't give in. It is like wearing a seat belt in the car: once children know it is a must, they will stop fighting. Remember, if you too wear a hat, the fight will be much easier.

There are three basic styles of hats we recommend for toddlers and young children.

Bucket hats. These hats are worn by all ages and are the most practical for sun protection. They are soft and crushable and come with a two-and-a-half- to three-inch brim. The hat protects the top of the head, the forehead, the tops of the ears, most of the back of the neck, and the cheeks. They come in small sizes for babies, with or without a cotton drawstring around the crown to adjust the size.

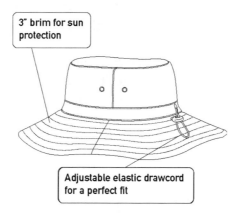

figure 13.1: Bucket Hat

Legionnaire (flappy-jack) hats. This is styled like a baseball cap but with a wider visor and a special neck protection flap. The hat protects the forehead, nose, ears, the back of the neck, the top of the head, and most of the cheeks. It is often seen as part of school uniforms for young children in Australia. These hats come in all sizes, including small sizes for babies, with or without cotton drawstrings.

Jennifer Lopez uses tanning sprays.

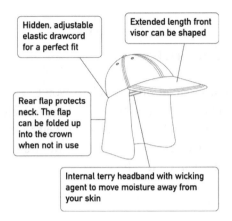

figure 13.2: Legionnaire Hat

Broadbrim hats. This hat is styled with a wide, floppy brim and is made from a soft material. It protects a baby's or toddler's head, forehead, nose, ears, neck, and sides of cheeks. This is sometimes the preferred hat for babies and toddlers because it is easy to fall asleep in. When children are older, this hat is appreciated for its durability. It can be crushed into backpacks or lunchboxes.

We do not believe hats for babies and toddlers should have a strap under the chin. While many manufacturers include them, we find they are uncomfortable for the child and prompt more resistance to wearing the hat. Some also argue that it is unsafe to have elastic or a cord around a child's neck.

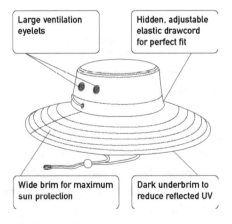

figure 13.3: Broadbrim Hat

Sun exposure causes premature aging.

Hats for Teenagers

We have learned the hard way that teenagers are the most unpredictable and sometimes defiant about what they will wear. We suggest that they choose from any of the adult sun protective hats we list, then decorate the hats to make them their own. We also encourage you to make sure they take a hat with them whenever they go to a sports activity, to camp, or to any outdoor gathering. Often, while they insist they won't need or wear a hat, they change their minds once they feel the sun.

Many teenage boys will argue that a baseball cap is enough protection. Remind them that it's not. Baseball caps provide no protection for the neck and ears and little protection for the cheeks, chin, and lips. However, since a baseball cap is probably better than no hat at all, sometimes it may be necessary to compromise, so long as a promise can be secured to use plenty of sunscreen.

Australian teenagers are now seen wearing hats. The once coveted tan is less fashionable, and the years of sun protection education in the schools are taking hold.

. . . .

Hats for All Ages

Following are descriptions of hats that offer excellent sun protection. When shopping for a hat, check the label to make sure the material is rated UPF 30, meaning that it will block 97 percent of UVR.

Crushable cotton or canvas hats. These hats usually have a three-inch brim. They are made from a thick cotton canvas that is lightweight and completely crushable. They are manufactured in numerous colors and in reversible styles, so they are highly appealing to girls. The brims turn up or down, and a scarf can be added for fashion. Women wear these hats for almost any outdoor activity: gardening, cookouts, painting, or walking. Leave one on the backseat of your car so you can grab it whenever you find yourself outside.

The skin is the largest organ in the human body.

Legionnaire hats. This hat offers the same high rate of protection as a child's legionnaire hat. It protects the top of the head; the ears, nose, and forehead; the back of the neck; and the cheeks. They are made in a range of natural and synthetic fabrics, some of which can be worn in or near the water. All legionnaire-style hats are easy to keep in a back-pack or on a boat and can be worn for almost any sport. Most recently, we have seen members of the University of Florida water polo team wearing them. The best legionnaire hats have elongated visors that are flexible enough to be custom shaped and protective neck flaps that are long enough to overlap the collar of a T-shirt. These are good hats to wear on a boat because the close-fitting cap does not easily blow off. You can buy them with clips that fasten the protective neck flap to the collar of your shirt to make sure they don't blow away.

Straw beach hats. These are cool, light, and comfortable, but they should be lined to provide the best UVR protection. Straw hats without lining offer inadequate protection. Straw hats should not be crushed, nor should they get wet. Straw beach hats should have a brim of three to five inches and should be rated to block 97 percent of UVR.

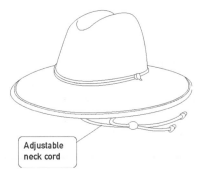

Adjustable neck cord

figure 13.4: Straw Beach Hat

Adult bucket hats. These have been worn by fishermen for many years. They are lightweight, crushable, and easy to wash and usually become an all-time favorite. For the best sun protection combined with comfort, find one that is made with a nylon microfiber that will

Women have a thicker hypodermis than men.

retain UVR protection even after extensive washing. These hats should have a brim of at least 3 inches.

Ventilated canvas hats. These hats have been popular for many years because they offer the coolness of airflow through ventilation. They can be shaped for a more formal style or used for any outside activity. For UVR protection, however, the ventilated fabric needs a lining that allows airflow, wicks away perspiration, and blocks UVR.

Broadbrim hats. These hats have a brim of three inches or more. For windy conditions, they usually have a drawstring to keep them in place. For the best sun protection, they will also have a dark underbrim to minimize reflected UVR. These hats offer protection for the entire face and are an excellent choice for garden work.

Sun hats. This versatile style is lightweight and can be used for most sports, including golfing, hiking, and tennis. It has a three-inch brim and is crushable for easy packing. If it is carefully made, it will include a headband on the inside to wick away moisture. Different manufacturers make it with different fabrics and features. Check the label to be sure it is easily washable.

Helmets. A sun protective fabric flap can be added to any helmet to protect the back of the neck. Helmets should be worn by people of any age during activities that could result in a head injury. Always wear sunscreen on your face when wearing a helmet.

· ·
School Policies Should Encourage the Use of Hats

For many years, school dress codes have prohibited the wearing of hats because of concerns regarding gang association or sloppy attire. To overcome this obstacle in California schools, state legislation was proposed by the Billy Foundation and introduced by Senator Don Perata to allow children to wear sun protective hats at recess and during sports. The bill became effective January 1, 2001. It was amended one

It is estimated that 23 percent of sun exposure happens during childhood (Godar 2001).

year later to allow sunscreen use at school. Its passage has prompted many California schools to revise their dress codes.

However, the fact remains that most schools still lack a comprehensive sun safety program. As we mentioned in chapter 8, excellent guidelines for school-based sun safety programs have been issued by various respected organizations, most notably the CDC. Now it is time for all schools to take action. Discuss hats and other sun safety issues with your child's principal, and lobby for meaningful policy implementation. Most of the SunSmart programs in Australia were the result of concerned parents encouraging schools to adopt sun protection programs.

Ongoing sun protection policies for children in Australia include the rule *No hat, no sun.* We would like to see a similar policy adopted by schools in this country. There are many positive outcomes of this message:

* Children learn early that they must protect themselves from UVR.

* Children learn that their parents and teachers are serious about protecting them.

* Parents learn that hats are one of the most important methods of sun protection.

* Children develop the habit of having a hat.

* Children know that the whole community supports the habit of wearing a hat.

You can find out more about developing comprehensive policy suggestions for schools in "Online Resources." You can also find an extensive list of hat retailers.

Photoaging occurs when UVR strikes the skin.

Summing Up

Be AWARE that wearing a hat is an essential method of sun protection. Hats are now designed to protect the entire head and neck and are made with fabrics that are lightweight, easy to care for, and rated to block up to 97 percent of UVR. Remember, however, that hats cannot provide full protection against indirect or reflected UVR and should always be worn with sunscreen and sunglasses.

Skin conditions associated with photoaging are
considered medical problems.

* 14 *

protecting your eyes
from the sun

Each year, over 300 million pairs of sunglasses are sold in the United States (USDHHS, FDA, CDRH 1998). That is over one pair for every man, woman, and child in the country! While all of these glasses will filter UVR to some degree, not all of them will protect your eyes.

Eyes need light to provide vision. Yet too much light will harm them. This is part of the paradox of our relationship with the sun. The American Academy of Ophthalmology has begun a campaign to educate the general public about the effect of photodamage to the eye. This damage includes macular degeneration, cataracts, and mela-noma of the retina. Further, the American Academy of Pediatrics Committee on Environmental Health (1999) recommends that infants and children wear sunglasses that block 99 percent of the full UV spectrum.

· ·

How Your Eyes Work

The eye is quite complex. It is composed of many layers, each serving a different purpose.

The outer layer consists of the tough but sensitive cornea and sclera. The *sclera* is the white of the eye, which protects it from injury or irritation. The *cornea*, an extension of the sclera at the front of the eye, acts as a transparent window through which light can pass. The cornea also covers and protects the *iris*, which is the colored part of the eye. The iris is where the most UVB rays are absorbed.

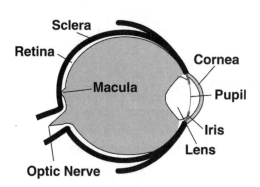

figure 14.1: Anatomy of the Eye

Studies have shown that the color of the iris does not provide protection against UVR. People used to believe that light-colored eyes were more susceptible to damage, but it is now known that brown eyes are 80 percent more likely to develop cataracts and two and a half times more likely to need surgery to treat problems related to UVR exposure (Younan et al. 2002).

The iris expands and contracts to widen or narrow the *pupil*. Together, they act like a sophisticated piece of machinery to allow for clear vision in all different lighting situations. When too much light is directed toward the eye, the pupil gets smaller, allowing only a narrow stream to pass through. When there is insufficient light, the pupil opens wide, admitting as much light as possible.

But the iris and the pupil are only part of the machine. Behind the pupil is the *lens*, which—when working properly—is so clear that light can pass right through it. The lens focuses the light passing though it by altering its shape. The *retina*, which is attached to the innermost lining of the eyeball, then receives the image that the lens and cornea have *refracted* or bent and sends it to the brain.

Severity of wrinkles depends largely on UVR exposure over a lifetime.

As with any machine, each part must be well maintained. In front of the lens is an area called the *anterior chamber,* which is filled with watery fluid that helps maintain the proper pressure inside the eye. The area behind the lens and in front of the retina is filled with a jellylike substance that is colorless and clear, called the *vitreous humor.*

All these different parts of the eye need to be working for vision to be clear.

Eye Problems Associated with UVR Exposure

Blinking and squinting are your eyes' only natural defenses to UVR damage, and they offer limited protection. UVR exposure can damage your eyes in various ways, including sunburn to the eyelids or eyes. Cataracts are the form of eye damage most often associated with chronic sun exposure. However, macular degeneration and melanoma of the eye are also commonly attributed to UVR damage.

Sunburn to the Eyes and Eyelids

The eyelid rarely gets burned, unless someone has fallen asleep in the sun, but individuals with a history of prolonged sun exposure are at risk of all three skin cancers—basal cell, squamous cell, and melanoma—on the eyelid.

"Snow blindness," a condition known medically as *ultraviolet keratoconjunctivitis,* is sunburn to the eyeball caused by the double whammy of direct UVR and reflected UVR from the snow. Snow blindness is a temporary condition. It is common to skiers and snowboarders as well as people who enjoy water sports, where UVR is reflected from the surface of the water.

Fortunately, snow blindness will usually heal itself. The eyelid reacts by closing involuntarily, and the person is "blind." It is an extremely painful condition, sometimes described as feeling like sandpaper is scraping your eyes, and it can be avoided by wearing goggles

Even if you already have damaged skin,
you will benefit from sun protection.

or sunglasses. There is little evidence that the damage to the cornea from snow blindness is permanent, but damage to the lens from chronic exposure is thought to lead to cataracts.

Cataracts

As you grow older, you may notice that your vision has become cloudy or that colors look dull. These may be symptoms of *cataracts*. Cataracts usually form in individuals middle-aged and older. The American Academy of Ophthalmology (2003) estimates that cataracts affect 60 percent of people older than sixty and that over 1.4 million cases are treated surgically every year in the United States, costing billions of dollars in medical care. While no one knows for sure what causes cataracts, most ophthalmologists believe that exposure to UVR plays a major contributing role.

Cataracts form when a change in the chemical composition of the lens creates a cloudy substance that becomes increasingly difficult to see through. While the chemical changes that create cataracts are sometimes related to a hereditary enzyme defect, a trauma to the eye, or diabetes, most often they are caused by chronic exposure to UVR. UVR exposure creates fragments called *free radicals* that appear to be the primary reason for the chemical change within the lens. UVB is thought to be most damaging because the lens absorbs these rays.

A study of fishermen found that those who developed cataracts had 20 percent more exposure to sunlight in every year of life (Taylor et al. 1988). The authors concluded that avoiding the sun between 10:00 A.M. and 4:00 P.M. and wearing a wide-brim hat and sunglasses could help prevent cataracts.

Symptoms

You may not even know you have cataracts if they form at the edge of the lens. However, cloudiness at the center of the lens will interfere with clear vision and will need treatment. Symptoms include the following:

* double or blurred vision

Daily moisturizers and makeup foundations should always have an SPF of 15 or higher.

* sensitivity to light and glare, possibly including halos around lights at night

* dull colors

* frequent changes in eyeglass prescriptions

* change in the color of the pupil, which is normally black, to yellow or white

Diagnosis

A diagnosis of cataracts can be made by a doctor using a handheld viewing instrument. An ophthalmologist should, however, determine the extent of the damage caused by the cataract with more extensive testing.

Treatment

If a cataract is diagnosed, the ophthalmologist will measure the shape, size, and general health of the eye to determine whether a lens implant will be effective. A lens implant is often the best option, because it will help restore good peripheral vision and depth perception with a minimum of magnification and distortion. In this procedure, the clouded lens is surgically removed and replaced with a plastic *intraocular lens*. This is an hour-long operation that often requires no hospitalization. Having a lens implant is, however, a serious procedure, and all risks should be discussed with your doctor.

Macular Degeneration

Macular degeneration is a physical disturbance or change at the center of the retina, in an area called the *macula*. The macula provides you with the ability to see details. You need it for reading and doing close-up work of any nature. Vision loss from macular degeneration usually occurs gradually and will typically affect both eyes but at different rates. The cause of macular degeneration is unknown, but it

The American Academy of Dermatology recommends that you apply sunscreen every day (AAD 2004a).

is generally agreed that UVR—particularly UVB—may accelerate the progression of the disease.

Advanced macular degeneration (AMD) is the leading cause of vision loss among Americans age sixty-five and over (Meadows 2002). The National Eye Institute (2004) estimated that 1.7 million Americans had some form of AMD, and since the number of Americans over the age of sixty-five is expected to double by 2030, this number is expected to grow. Women tend to be at greater risk for AMD than men, and whites are much more likely to lose vision from AMD than blacks.

There are two forms of the disease. About 85 percent of people have what's known as the "dry" type, and the remainder have the "wet" type, which is more severe. In the dry type, the light-sensitive vision cells deteriorate, but there is no bleeding. In the wet type of AMD, blood vessels behind the retina grow under the macula and may leak blood and fluid.

Symptoms

Ophthalmologists recommend that you make an appointment immediately if you experience any of the following:

* Distortion of straight lines or distortion at the center of vision

* A dark, blurry, or "washed-out" area in the center of vision

* Reduction or change in color perception

Diagnosis

Your ophthalmologist may be the first to find indications of macular degeneration during a routine exam. Declining vision or the formation of new vessels will alert your doctor to the possibility.

The American Academy of Dermatology recommends that you reapply sunscreen every two hours or after swimming or perspiring (AAD 2004a).

Treatment

Early detection is important because your eyes can sometimes be treated before symptoms appear, and this may delay or reduce the severity of the disease. At this time, there is no known cure for the disease.

Melanoma of the Eye

Like melanoma found anywhere on the body, melanoma of the eye may be the direct result of UVR exposure. The tumor that is found in the eye may be the primary site of the cancer, or it may be that the cancer has spread to the eye from another location in the body. Either way, the melanoma is likely to have been started by the biological reaction of the body to UVR. A melanoma tumor will eventually cause retinal detachment and distortion of vision.

Symptoms

Unfortunately, unlike melanomas found on the skin, melanoma of the eye may not have any early symptoms. However, because melanomas are found increasingly as people age, a regular eye exam may be the best way to detect the disease.

If you experience any of the following symptoms, contact your ophthalmologist immediately:

* red, painful eye

* small defect on the iris or *conjunctiva* (the mucous membrane protecting the ball of the eye and the inner surface of the eyelids)

* change in the color of the iris

* poor vision in one eye

* bulging eyes

There are many ways to repair damaged skin, from lotions to lasers.

Diagnosis

An eye examination with an *ophthalmoscope* (a handheld instrument used to examine the internal portion of the eye) reveals a single round or oval lump within the eye. Among other tests that may be given, an ultrasound exam will determine the size of the tumor and the exact location, a cranial scan will determine if the tumor has spread, and a skin biopsy will be done if there is an affected area on the skin.

Treatment

Melanoma of the eye is treated differently depending on the diagnosis. A small melanoma may be removed with a laser or with radiation therapy. Chemotherapy may be needed if the tumor has spread. Surgical removal of the eye may be necessary to prevent the cancer from spreading. In most cases, there is a 60 to 80 percent chance of survival for at least five years from the time of diagnosis. If the cancer has spread, the survival rate is much lower.

Taking Care of Your Eyes

Having regular eye exams is an important part of taking care of your eyes. Below we have listed the guidelines established by the American Academy of Ophthalmology (2004). We recommend you contact this organization if you need to find an eye doctor in your area (see "Online Resources").

Recommended Guidelines for Eye Exams

Through age five. Infants from newborn to three months should be checked for diseases of the eye, and they should be checked again at six months. Toddlers at age three should be screened for common childhood problems such as nearsightedness and farsightedness. At age

People with a family history of skin cancer should routinely have body checks.

five, children should be checked again. Poor eyesight can cause slowness in early childhood development.

Puberty to age thirty-nine. In this age range, you should be checked if you experience any eye problems or visual changes such as pain, floaters, flashes of light, blurry vision, or eye injury. Most people have healthy eyes during this time, although many need corrective prescriptions.

Ages forty to sixty-five. In this age range, you should be examined every two to four years. People at higher risk for eye diseases need to be examined more often. For example, adults with diabetes should have yearly eye exams. Other people at higher risk include African-Americans over age forty, people with a family history of eye disease, or those with a history of eye injury.

Over age sixty-five. In this age range, you should be examined every one to two years.

Your eyes, like your skin, should be protected from UVR from the day you are born. Babies under the age of six months should be kept out of the sun completely. As we mentioned earlier, the American Academy of Pediatrics recommends the use of sunglasses for infants and children.

Sunglasses should be worn by people of all ages to protect the eyes when outside. Close-fitting, wraparound glasses offer the best protection. Further, a hat with a three-inch brim blocks direct UVR rays from your eyes.

. . . .
Choosing Sunglasses

That an estimated 300 million sunglasses are distributed each year in this country is, in many ways, good news. It means the public is taking positive steps to protect their eyes from the harmfulness of UVR.

Sun protective clothing should have hangtags indicating testing standards.

However, when you buy sunglasses, it is important that you know how to identify glasses that best block UVA and UVB.

In the United States, nonprescription sunglasses are regulated as medical devices by the Center for Devices and Radiological Health in the FDA. However, there are hundreds of manufacturers, importers, and distributors, and the standards and labeling regarding UVR protection are voluntary.

So how do you, the consumer, know that these standards are being met, and how do you know what they mean with regard to safely protecting your eyes? If you are aware of the following few facts, you will likely be able to choose sunglasses that will adequately protect your eyes:

* All sunglasses filter UVR to some degree, but not all sunglasses offer the same UVR protection. The best protection is offered by glasses that block UVA and UVB rays between 280 and 400 nanometers. If standards have been met, one of the following codes will likely be listed on the label:

   ANSI Z80.3—1996, Ophthalmic—Nonprescription Sunglasses and Fashion Eyewear Requirements

   ISO 8980-3, Ophthalmic Optics—Uncut Finished Spectacle Lenses—Part 3—Transmittance Specification and Test Methods

   ISO 14889, Ophthalmic Optics—Spectacle Lenses —Fundamental Requirements for Uncut Finished Lenses

   ISO 10993, Biological Evaluation of Medical Devices—Parts 1 through 12

* Sunglasses with lens tints that are too light will not block glare. Pink, blue, or purple tints are purely cosmetic and are poor light blockers.

* The lens tint should be uniform, not streaked or with dark or light spots.

Ordinary moles are round or oval.

* The frame should fit comfortably on your face and not too tightly over your ears. Wraparound frames offer the best UVR protection.

* All sunglasses must be impact resistant, but they are not shatterproof. They should not be used for high-impact sports or industrial safety purposes unless they are specifically designed for these uses.

* Sunglasses cannot protect against intense light sources, such as sunlamps, lasers, welding torches, or solar eclipses. Special lenses are made for these conditions that meet different standards. Be careful not to use regular sunglasses if you are exposed to these light sources.

One concern that has often been voiced and was recently discredited is the idea that pupil dilation from wearing sunglasses can cause problems for the eyes. Gies, Roy, and Elliott (1990) suggest that there is very minimal dilation of the pupil when wearing sunglasses and that the effectiveness of sunglasses in protecting the eyes against UVB radiation far outweighs concern about dilation.

Shades and Tints

Sunglass lenses come in different shades and colors. (A treated clear lens will block UVR, but be sure to check that it blocks both UVB and UVA.) So how do you know if one color is better than another? An easy rule to remember is that light to medium shades are good for daily wear, but for bright conditions, outdoor sports, boating, and some driving, darker shades are appropriate.

Always check the label or tag to find out how much UVR will be blocked; a good standard to look for is 99.5 percent. Also check how much visible light will be blocked, to ensure the sunglasses are safe for driving. Some tints can block the true colors of traffic lights. You should not wear sunglasses while driving at night.

Ordinary moles have a sharp, even border with the skin.

The following tint guide may help you choose the best sunglasses for different activities. These tints are also used for goggles.

* Gray does not enhance contrast, nor does it distort color perception. It is good for golf, cycling, or running.

* Green provides fair contrast in low light and helps reduce eyestrain in bright light. It is good for driving and most outdoor activities.

* Brown enhances contrast. It is good for hazy days or when there is glare from surfaces such as water or snow—sailing, fishing, skiing, or playing tennis.

* Amber helps to minimize eyestrain by providing contrast in bright conditions. It is good for pilots, hang gliders, and skiers.

* Yellow is best for overcast days or when there is low light.

* Vermilion (red) enhances the contrast of objects against blue (sky) and green backgrounds. It is good for skiers.

Types of Sunglasses

There is no end to the types of sunglasses that are available. We have tried to narrow down the categories to provide descriptions of what you can expect. Always check the labels to be sure the sunglasses block 99.5 percent UVR—both UVA and UVB—and be sure the fit is right for you.

Ordinary moles are a uniform brown in color.

Children's Sunglasses

Children, including infants, should wear sunglasses routinely whenever they go outside. If you make sure of this, they will wear them as easily as a seat belt in a car—no questions asked.

Children generally like the idea of sunglasses, particularly because there are so many great designs and colors available. Wraparounds are the most protective because they shield the eyes from UVR coming from all directions. Plastic frames are the most durable (although they can break and the lenses may pop out of the frame), and there are accessories that make wearing them easier. Sunglass cords, which come in a multitude of colors, will help keep them from getting lost. Hard cases keep them from scratching when thrown in a backpack, and a cleaning cloth gets rid of smudgy fingerprints. Oval, round, rectangular, and geometric shapes are all popular and can be found at specialty stores like Sunglass Hut or optical chain stores like Pearle Vision and LensCrafters.

Prescription Sunglasses

Prescription sunglasses are manufactured as medical devices and are therefore the most trustworthy for blocking harmful UVR. They can be made for almost anyone who wears prescription glasses or contact lenses. They are available in basic, bifocal, and progressive lens options, and they come in nearly every sunglass design with the exception of wraparound (because the curves distort vision). Most optical shops make prescription sunglasses attractive by offering special discounts on a second pair of glasses.

Keep in mind that *photochromic* lenses—those that darken in the sunlight and become much lighter indoors—usually do not have UVR protection built into the lenses. You must specify that you want the additional UVR coating applied to the lens to have this protection.

Performance and Sports Sunglasses

Manufacturers have developed lightweight, flexible, and durable materials to be used for the most competitive or casual sports. While many people believe the most important aspect of these glasses is the

Ordinary moles are less than a quarter of an inch in diameter.

optical quality and visual enhancement provided by the lenses, we believe that protecting eyes from UVR problems such as snow blindness makes sunglasses an essential part of any athlete's gear.

Polycarbonate lenses are popular for sports sunglasses because they are strong and impact resistant. Most people shy away from glass lenses for sports eyewear, but they do have great optical quality.

Polarized Sunglasses

Polarized lenses are primarily used for their ability to block glare from surfaces like sand or water by absorbing light that scatters in all but one direction—the vertical plane. While polarizing has nothing to do with blocking UVR, these glasses also contain UVR-blocking chemicals and offer excellent protection.

Polarized sunglasses are used for driving—to reduce the glare from roads—and by fishermen, boaters, skiers, golfers, bikers, and joggers. They are also used by people recovering from eye surgery and by those troubled by glare from computer screens. They are available for bifocal, progressive, photochromic, and single-vision lenses.

Fashion Sunglasses

Sunglasses have become fashion accessories. You can find almost any major designer name with a line of sunglasses, and you can spend any amount of money for the pleasure of wearing them. Most lenses in designer glasses clearly meet standards and are good choices for sun protection. However, it is up to you as the consumer to be aware of the pitfalls. Some designs are simply too small to offer UVR protection, many don't offer wraparound protection, and some can't be worn during sporting activities. If you choose designer sunglasses, choose only those that offer good UVR protection.

Fit

Finally, when shopping for sunglasses, remember that if the frame does not fit comfortably to your face, you probably won't wear

Ordinary moles that are raised are always dome-shaped.

them. Frames can be adjusted. Metal frames normally have screws that can be tightened. Some plastic frames can be heated slightly and formed, but we suggest you try to avoid this. Try the glasses on carefully before buying them. If you buy from one of the many optical stores, you can ask to have the frames adjusted while you are there.

Summing Up

Be AWARE of the need to protect your eyes from ultraviolet radiation. Brown eyes are damaged by the sun as easily as blue eyes or hazel eyes. Sun-damaged eyes can develop several diseases, including cataracts, macular degeneration, and melanoma of the eye. Children, including infants, should wear sunglasses—along with a hat with a three-inch brim—to provide the best protection for their eyes. Quality sunglass lenses will block at least 99.5 percent of UVR.

Aldara (imiquimod) has been approved by the FDA for use on superficial basal cell carcinoma.

protecting yourself using shade

Throughout the book, we have stated that it's important to avoid unprotected exposure to the sun between the hours of 10:00 A.M. and 4:00 P.M. While avoiding the sun is best achieved by staying indoors, this is not realistic. This chapter discusses some of the ways you can help protect yourself by using shade. We describe what makes shade effective, and we list ways to create shade. While some shade is always better than no shade, it does not actually provide 100 percent protection. So be AWARE of all methods of sun protection and use them in combination with seeking shade.

Why Shade Isn't Always Enough

Finding effective shade is not always as simple as sitting in the shadow of a tree or a beach umbrella. UVR is reflected by many surfaces, and while direct UVR travels in a straight line through the atmosphere, indirect UVR may come from any direction.

Snow, water, sand, and concrete reflect UVR. Less obvious indirect UVR would be reflected from a building, particularly a building painted white. Given that UVR does bounce, while you are sitting under a tree next to a beautiful lake or under the beach umbrella on a lovely sandy beach, you may still be exposed to enough indirect UVR to get sunburned. It will take longer to get burned than when you are directly exposed, but the consequences are the same.

Gies and colleagues (1999) measured how much exposure two subjects received while participating in different outdoor activities. They compared a picnicker in the shade of a tree to a walker, who was predominately in the open. As expected, the walker's exposure was greater because there was nothing blocking either direct or indirect UVR. However, sitting under foliage (in shade), the picnicker had lower, but still constant, exposure to UVR. The explanation was found in the indirect UVR—the UVR reflected from the ground, dust particles, or perhaps nearby water. The findings make it clear that while shade is an important method of sun protection, it does not provide complete protection from ambient exposure and should be used in combination with other methods.

. . . .
Providing Shade

We hope that as more people understand the health risks of sun exposure, there will be a cultural shift toward providing shade in public areas. In Australia, sun protection is considered a social responsibility. Accordingly, schools, state and local governments, and the federal government work together to provide protection. The provision of shade structures is best addressed by local groups, although national architectural organizations should address standards.

Locally, shade should be provided for public areas such as beaches, bike paths, parking lots, childcare centers, roadside lookouts, outdoor dining facilities, parks, playgrounds, public docks, shopping malls, fairgrounds, sporting fields, and swimming pools. Every city and county should take a close look at all public areas and be sure effective shading is provided. Guidelines are available from organizations such as state architectural boards and the U.S. General Services Administration (see "Online Resources").

People with more than fifty moles may have a higher chance
of getting melanoma.

In this section, we'll talk about how you can purchase or design shade structures to protect yourself and others effectively.

What to Consider When Constructing or Designing Shade

Both time of day and nearby reflective surfaces must be considered when planning shade.

Time of day. If you are planning the placement of a structure for shade, you need to understand the sun's path. For example, it would be pointless to provide overhead shade for an audience watching a soccer game at 3:00 P.M. or to place an awning over a window that gets only northeastern exposure. To accurately predict the behavior of shade provided by solid objects, you need to know the direction the shadow will fall and the length it will be at different times of day and different times of year.

Surfaces that reflect UVR. Knowing which surfaces reflect UVR will help you better assess the level of indirect UVR exposure from surrounding surfaces and choose a shade structure that blocks reflected UVR. Sliney (1986) lists common materials that reflect UVR and the percentage of the total ambient UVR each reflects:

* white house paint (22 percent)

* dry beach sand (15 to 18 percent)

* light-colored concrete (8 to 12 percent)

* asphalt road (4 to 9 percent)

* open water (3 to 8 percent)

* lawn grass (2 to 5 percent)

There are four basic types of melanoma.

Effective Shade Structures

Effective shade works to block both direct and indirect exposure to UVR. Here are guidelines you can use to seek the best UVR protection available:

* Shade structures with solid sides are best for blocking both direct and indirect UVR.

* Shade structures made from solid materials have the highest UPF ratings.

* Shade structures that are located amongst foliage are more protective than foliage alone.

There are countless ways to provide shade. Here are a few of the most popular.

Trees

Trees are often the first choice for shade. They help improve the environment, are beautiful to look at, and can last for generations. Selecting trees for shade does require some research, however, and decisions should be made carefully. So do your homework—make sure the tree you select will provide thick foliage and will grow trouble-free in the area you select. Here are a few general guidelines for selecting and planting shade trees:

* Choose the location to maximize shade. For the best shade, plant on the western and southern sides of a building. In especially warm parts of the country, you may also want to plant on the southeastern side of the building, since late morning sun is often very hot.

* Make sure you do a site analysis. This should include seasonal temperature information, humidity, sunlight, and expected adverse weather conditions. It should also include a description of the type of soil and how

Nonmelanoma skin cancer is the most common cancer among Caucasians in the United States.

much water it contains. And don't forget to find out if there are any root obstructions such as rocks, utility lines, or septic tanks. Soil testing and a visual examination of the site will help you choose wisely and avoid future problems.

* Choose trees that have wide-spreading, dense leaf canopies.

* Know what kind of plants you may have under the shade, because they will be affected by the density of the tree's foliage.

* Plant trees in clusters to provide the most effective shade cover as well as create interesting patterns.

* Make sure the trees you select do not have canopies that grow too low or too high, blocking vision or creating safety problems.

Never rely solely on tree shade for sun protection. Trees can help keep your house cool and can provide some protection from UVR exposure, but because UV rays bounce from the ground and the side of the house, you should always wear sun protective clothing and sunscreen while enjoying the shade of a tree.

Shade Sails

Shade sails are used throughout Australia in schoolyards, parks, campgrounds, backyards, and anywhere else natural shade is lacking. Shade sails can be used almost anywhere because they can be attached to an existing structure or to posts. They are usually made of a high-density polyethylene cloth that is specially manufactured with tensioned fabric structures in mind.

There are some drawbacks to shade sails, however. Because they act as a roof with no sides, they block only direct UVR, not reflected UVR, and give a false sense of security. Further, while the tight weave can absorb up to 98 percent of direct UVR, it may lose its

Our analysis shows that sun protective clothing sales are three times sunscreen sales in Australia.

protective abilities when stretched or washed. Color also determines the effectiveness of shade sails, with darker colors being more effective.

Shade sails are an important method of providing shade, but you should still wear sun protective clothing and sunscreen.

Awnings

Awnings over windows, particularly windows facing west or south, cut down on heat levels in the interior of buildings and block UVR. Window awnings that are made from solid roofing materials provide the highest UVR protection. However, most window awnings are made from canvaslike materials, and the UVR protection level will depend on the tightness of the weave, color, and wear. Look for material that has double-sided color and a coat of acrylic to repel water. Some companies have materials independently tested for UVA and UVB protection levels. We recommend you look for a UPF of 50 or higher for any awning material.

Umbrellas and Canopies

Umbrellas can be an especially helpful method of sun protection. Stashed in a purse, briefcase, or in the car, umbrellas can be used as an alternative to a hat and can provide instant shade. Like anything made with fabric, however, umbrellas and canopies provide different levels of protection depending on the type of material used. The denser the weave, the higher the UVR protection. If the material is plastic coated, it will provide better protection, because plastics generally absorb UVR. Look for labels indicating UPF ratings. While UPF rating is not required in this country, you will find several sun protection companies that offer products made from tested materials.

Umbrellas and canopies do not protect against indirect UVR exposure, so sun protective clothing and sunscreen should still be worn.

Melanoma originates in the melanocytes in the skin.

·
Glass Tinting and Films

Glass tinting and films are important ways to reduce exposure to UVR. Two types of glass—auto and building—are the primary focus of the glass tinting and film industry. We look at each to determine its effectiveness in reducing UVR exposure.

Auto Glass Tinting

While a car provides substantial shading, the glass areas do not block UVR exposure. Since it is not uncommon for people to spend several hours a day in a car, the implications for skin problems are considerable. In the United States, where the steering wheel is on the left side of the car, photoaging and skin cancers likely have a higher rate of occurrence on the left arm, left hand, left side of the face and neck, and left ear. The opposite side will be affected in Australia or England. Further, damage to the eyes from glare and direct UVR increases the more people drive.

There are federal and state laws regarding glass tinting for automobiles. It is hard to know, however, whether these laws have been formulated with attention to the potential danger of UVR exposure. Many laws apparently consider heat, privacy, and safety, but we have not found direct discussion of sunburn or skin cancers.

Under federal laws, a vehicle's driver-side and passenger-side windows may only be legally tinted up to 70 percent *visual light transmission,* or VLT. This is the normal factory tint most new cars come equipped with. The higher the VLT, the more light will shine through the film.

Individual states can set their own guidelines for other windows, and these guidelines vary greatly. For example, New Hampshire does not allow front side windows to be tinted at all but allows a 35 percent VLT on rear side windows. North Carolina allows passenger cars to have 35 percent VLT on both driver- and passenger-side windows, as well as on the rear window.

Wearing a hat will help prevent sun damage to the eyes and face.

There are safety concerns about using window tint in cars. The tint can be reflective, which is dangerous to other drivers, and it can be hard to see through at night. However, we believe the government needs to restudy the issue with regard to sun protection and find a tint that will protect drivers and passengers from UVR.

Gies, Roy, and Zongli (1992) studied the solar UVR levels inside an automobile. Their findings confirm that tinting the glass on automobiles would significantly reduce people's exposure to UVR, especially UVA. The authors also warned that careful consideration should be given to the effect the tints had on the color perception and reaction times of drivers.

Several tints are available that provide sufficient protection while still allowing full visibility in various driving conditions, including darkness. The Skin Cancer Foundation recommends UVShield (see "Online Resources") because it meets the following criteria:

* legal for application on car windows in all fifty states

* approved for application to car windshields with a physician's prescription (contact your local department of motor vehicles)

* offers 99.9 percent protection against UVA and UVB

Window Tinting and Window Films for the Home

The use of glass in the average home, expressed as a percentage of the total wall space, has grown from about 7 percent in the 1930s to 20 percent today and is still growing. Over the same period, the average home has grown from 1,100 square feet to 2,150 square feet. The combination means homes have a lot of glass and a lot of UVR exposure (Kubler 1999).

UVR exposure in the home is primarily responsible for the fading of fabrics, carpets, wallpapers, woods, antiques, and artworks. But more importantly, UVR exposure in the home has recently been associated with premature aging of the skin and some skin cancers. Sun

More than 55,000 Americans were diagnosed with melanoma in 2004 (AAD 2004c).

sensitive people especially are at risk of exposure to direct and indirect UVA from windows. UVA rays penetrate glass directly into a room and can bounce further into the interior. In an effort to protect themselves, many sun sensitive people block windows with heavy fabrics and lose the benefit of light.

UVR protective films for windows can nearly eliminate these two sets of problems. The latest development in window films is the introduction of films that protect against 99.9 percent of UVR. This is the highest degree of UVR protection available in the window film market and is—practically speaking—as close to total protection as possible.

Vista Window Film carries the Skin Cancer Seal of Recommendation and has been recommended by physicians nationwide as an effective preventative measure for patients with solar sensitivity, sun-related diseases, and skin cancers.

Summing Up

Protecting yourself from UVR means giving careful consideration to the environment in which you live and work. Providing areas of shade—effective shade that blocks direct and indirect UVR—where you and your family can find shelter is an important method of sun protection and part of being AWARE.

Taking responsibility for UVR exposure in your car and in your house can be difficult and expensive. However, once you know the facts, you can use them to talk to your state representative about automobile glass standards. You can also make better decisions about tinting or films for your home windows.

Sunburns at any time throughout life can cause skin cancer.

be AWARE

We have studied the advice given by countless organizations, discussed it with experts around the world, and summarized it in the following acronym. We believe this is the most up-to-date advice about sun protection and is the best way to summarize all the information in this book.

Be AWARE that exposure to UVR can cause premature aging of the skin and skin cancers, including melanoma.

A—avoid unprotected exposure at any time but especially during the hours of peak ultraviolet radiation (between 10:00 A.M. and 4:00 P.M.)

W—wear sun protective clothing, including a long-sleeve shirt, a hat with a three-inch brim, and sunglasses, and seek shade

A—apply broad-spectrum sunscreen with a sun protection factor (SPF) of 30 or higher to all unprotected skin twenty minutes before exposure and reapply every two hours while exposed

R—routinely check your whole body for changes in your skin and report suspicious changes to a physician

E—express the need for sun protection to your family and community

online resources

Federal Government Agencies

Cancer Information Service
  http://cis.nci.nih.gov

Centers for Disease Control and Prevention
  www.cdc.gov

Department of Health and Human Services
  www.os.dhhs.gov

Environmental Protection Agency
  www.epa.gov

Food and Drug Administration
  www.fda.gov

National Aeronautics and Space Administration (NASA)
  www.nasa.gov

National Cancer Institute
  www.nci.nih.gov

National Institute of Arthritis and Musculoskeletal and Skin Diseases
  www.niams.nih.gov

National Institute on Aging
  www.nia.nih.gov

National Institutes of Health
www.nia.nih.gov

National Library of Medicine
www.nlm.nih.gov

U.S. General Services Administration
www.gsa.gov

. . . .

National Organizations and Foundations

AMC Cancer Research Center
www.amc.org

American Academy of Dermatology
www.aad.org

American Academy of Facial Plastic and Reconstructive Surgery
www.aafprs.com

American Academy of Family Physicians
www.aafp.org

American Academy of Ophthalmology
www.aao.org

American Academy of Pediatrics
www.aap.org

American Association for Health Education
www.aahperd.org/aahe

American Board of Medical Specialties
www.abms.org

American Cancer Society
www.cancer.org

American Melanoma Foundation
www.melanomafoundation.org

American Pharmacists Association
www.aphanet.org

American Public Health Association
www.apha.org

Wearing sunglasses that block UVA and UVB can reduce your risk of
melanoma of the eye.

American School Health Association
www.ashaweb.org

American Society of Plastic Surgeons
www.plasticsurgery.org

Billy Foundation
www.bfmelanoma.com

Cancer Care
cancercare.org

Cancer Research and Prevention Foundation
www.preventcancer.org

Dermatology Nurses' Association
www.dna.inurse.com

Melanoma International Foundation
www.melanomaintl.org

Melanoma Research Foundation
www.melanoma.org

National Association of School Nurses
www.nasn.org

National Council on Skin Cancer Prevention
www.skincancerprevention.org

National Safety Council
www.nsc.org

Skin Cancer Foundation
www.skincancer.org

. . . .

Melanoma Information Sites

Most of the sites listed above will have general information about melanoma. More specific information can be found at the following:

American Academy of Dermatology
www.aad.org

American Melanoma Foundation
www.melanomafoundation.org

Skin cancer is the most common form of cancer in the United States.

Cancer Care
www.cancercare.org

Melanoma Patients' Information Page
www.mpip.org

Oncolink
www.oncolink.upenn.edu

Skin Cancer Foundation
www.skincancer.org

Skin Cancer Resources Directory
www.cancerindex.org/clinks2s.htm

· ·

Information about Medications That Cause Sun Sensitivity

American Pharmacists Association
www.aphanet.org

Medicine Net
www.medicinenet.com

· ·

Australian Organizations

ARPANSA
www.arpansa.gov.au

Australasian College of Dermatologists
www.dermcoll.asn.au

Australian Institute of Health and Welfare
www.aihw.gov.au

Cancer Council of South Australia
www.cancersa.org.au

Cancer Council Victoria
www.accv.org.au

Cancer Council Australia
www.cancer.org.au

Some medications may increase sun sensitivity.

Cancer Council of New South Wales
www.nswcc.org.au

Cancer Council of Western Australia
www.cancerwa.asn.au

Queensland Cancer Fund
www.qldcancer.com.au

....

Sun Protection Education for Children

ABCs for Fun in the Sun
www.aad.org/public/Publications/pamphlets/SunProtection
Children.html

Billy Foundation
www.bfmelanoma.com

Children's Sun Protection Program
www.skincancer.org/children

Choose Your Cover
www.cdc.gov/chooseyourcover

Kids' Connection
http://www.aad.org/public/Parentskids/kids.htm

National Council on Skin Cancer Prevention
www.skincancerprevention.org

Sun Protection: A Primary Teaching Resource
www.who.int/uv/publications/en/primaryteach.pdf

Sun Protection and Schools: How to Make a Difference
www.who.int/entity/uv/publications/en/sunprotschools.pdf

Sun Safety Alliance
www.sunsafetyalliance.org

Sun Safety for Kids
www.sunsafetyforkids.org

SunGuard Man Online
www.sunguardman.org

Elevation can play a role in increasing your risk of skin cancer.

SunSafe Project
www.dartmouth.edu/dms/sunsafe

SunSmart Campaign (Australia)
www.sunsmart.com.au

SunWise School Program
www.epa.gov/sunwise

Sunwise Stampede
www.foundation.sdsu.edu/sunwisestampede

. . . .

Sun Protection Education for Outdoor Workers

Solar Safe
http://ohp.ksc.nasa.gov/policies/pdf/SolarSafeProgram.pdf

Sun Sense: Laborers' Health and Safety Fund of North America
www.lhsfna.org

The Pocket Card
http://www.osha.gov/Publications/osha3166.pdf

The Sun Safety Kit
www.dhs.ca.gov/ps/cdic/CPNS/skin

Workplace Ultraviolet Radiation Protection
www.sunsmart.com.au

. . . .

UV Index Sites and Information

Climate Prediction Center of the National Weather Service
iwin.nws.noaa.gov/iwin/us/ultraviolet.html

Environmental Protection Agency (search by zip code)
www.epa.gov/sunwise/uvindex.html

National Weather Service: UV Index for 58 Cities
www.cpc.ncep.noaa.gov/products/stratosphere/uv_index/
uv_ annual.html

World Health Organization
www.who.int/uv/publications/en/Intersunguide.pdf

Early detection and treatment cures 95 percent of diagnosed basal cell and squamous cell skin cancers (AAD 2004c).

Sun Protective Clothing Companies

Coolibar
www.coolibar.com

Solar Eclipse
www.solareclipse.com

SolarVeil
www.solarveil.com

Sun Precautions
www.sunprecautions.com

Sun Protected
www.sunprotected.com

Sun Protective Clothing Company Ltd.
www.sunprotectiveclothing.com

Sun Solutions
www.sunsolutionsclothing.com

SunGrubbies
www.sungrubbies.com

Hat Resources (provided by Sun Safety for Kids)

Coolibar
www.coolibar.com

Dorfman Pacific (wholesale only)
www.dorfman-pacific.com

Radicool
www.radicoolaustralia.com

School Sun Hats
www.schoolsunhats.com

Skin Savers
www.skin-savers.com

Melanoma is a life-threatening illness.

Solar Eclipse
www.solareclipse.com

Solartex
www.solartex.com

Sun Safe
www.sunsafe.com

Sunday Afternoons
www.sundayafternoons.com

SunGrubbies
www.sungrubbies.com

Tilley Endurables
www.tilley.com

. . . .

Shade Resources

UVShield
www.uv-shield.com

Vista Window Film
www.vista-films.com

People prone to moles should protect themselves from UVR.

references

AAD. *See* American Academy of Dermatology.

AAD and CDC. *See* American Academy of Dermatology and Centers for Disease Control.

AAP. *See* American Academy of Pediatrics.

AAPCEH. *See* American Academy of Pediatrics Committee on Environmental Health.

ACS. *See* American Cancer Society.

AIHW and AACR. *See* Australian Institute of Health and Welfare and Australasian Association of Cancer Registries.

AMF. *See* American Melanoma Foundation.

American Academy of Dermatology. 1999a. The American Academy of Dermatology is concerned about FDA cap on sunscreens. *Press Release,* www.aad.org/PressReleases/concern.html.

———. 1999b. Vitiligo. *Public Resource Center,* http://www.aad.org/public/Publications/pamphlets/Vitiligo.htm

———. 2000a. Basal cell carcinoma. *Public Resource Center,* www.aad.org/public/Publications/pamphlets/BasalCellCarcinoma.htm

———. 2000b. Mature skin. *Public Resource Center,* www.aad.org/public/Publications/pamphlets/MatureSkin.htm.

———. 2000c. Squamous cell carcinoma. *Public Resource Center,* www.aad.org/public/Publications/pamphlets/SquamousCellCarcinoma.htm

———. 2000d. Sun protection for children. *Public Resource Center,* www.aad.org/public/Publications/pamphlets/SunProtectionChildren.htm

———. 2001. Basal cell carcinoma. Publication ID no. PAM51-6/03.

———. 2003. Fact sheet: Actinic keratoses and skin cancer. *Public Resource Center,* www.aad.org/public/News/DermInfo/ActKerSkCancerFAQ.htm.

———. 2004a. Facts about sunscreen. *Newsroom,* www.aad.org/aad/Newsroom/factsunscreen.htm.

———. 2004b. Melanoma fact sheet. *Public Resource Center,* www.aad.org/public/News/DermInfo/2004MelanomaFaq.htm.

———. 2004c. Skin cancer fact sheet. *Newsroom,* www.aad.org/aad/Newsroom/skincancerfact.htm.

American Academy of Dermatology and Centers for Disease Control. 1996. Significant knowledge gaps about melanoma skin cancer. *Morbidity and Mortality Weekly Report* 45 (RR-9): 1–41.

American Academy of Ophthalmology. 2003. Cataracts. *Medical Library,* www.aao.org.

———. 2004. Public Information. *Medem,* www.aao.org/aao/public.

American Academy of Pediatrics. 2004. Summer safety tips. *Health Topics,* www.aap.org.

American Academy of Pediatrics Committee on Environmental Health. 1999. Ultraviolet light: A hazard to children. *Pediatrics* 104 (2): 328–33.

American Cancer Society. 2003. Skin cancer facts. *Prevention and Early Detection,* www.cancer.org.

———. 2003b. Overview: Skin cancer—Melanoma. What causes melanoma skin cancer? *Cancer Topics,* www.cancer.org.

———. 2004a. Cancer facts and figures. www.cancer.org.

———. 2004b. Detailed guide: Skin cancer—Melanoma, What are the risk factors for melanoma? *Cancer Reference Information,* www.cancer.org.

———. 2004c. Detailed guide: Skin cancer—Nonmelanoma, What are the risk factors for nonmelanoma skin cancer. *Cancer Reference Information,* www.cancer.org.

American Melanoma Foundation. 2004. Skin cancer fact sheet. *Prevention,* melanomafoundation.org.

Australian Institute of Health and Welfare and Australasian Association of Cancer Registries. 2000. Cancer in Australia 1997: Incidence and mortality data for 1997 and selected data for 1998 and 1999. AIHW cat. no. Can 10. Canberra: AIHW (Cancer Series no. 15).

Autier, P., J. Dore, F. Lejuene, K. Koelmel, O. Geffeler, P. Hille, J. Cesarini, D. Lienard, A. Liabeuf, M. Joarlette, P. Chemaly, K. Hakim, A. Koeln, and U. Kleeberg. 1994. Cutaneous malignant melanoma and exposure to sunlamps or sunbeds: An EORTC multicenter case-control study in Belgium, France, and Germany. *International Journal of Cancer* 58:809–13.

Ayoub, J., The Skin Cancer Foundation. 2004. Telephone conversation with the authors, October 15.

Beddingfield, F., P. Cinar, S. Litwack, A. Ziogas, T. Taylor, and H. Anton-Culver. 2002. Gender- and age-specific differences in melanoma incidences. In *Melanoma: A Decision Analysis to Estimate the Effectiveness and Cost-Effectiveness of Screening and an Analysis of Relevant Epidemiology.* www.rand.org/publications/RGSD/RGSD167/RGSD167.ch3.pdf.

Brewster, B. 1997. Lifeguard skin cancer protection: An approach to protecting health and promoting image. Paper delivered to the International Life Saving Federation, International Medical/Rescue Conference, September.

Buller, D., A. Geller, M. Cantor, M. Buller, K. Rosseel, D. Hufford, L. Benjes, and R. Lew. 2002. Sun protection policies and environmental features in U.S. elementary schools. *Archives of Dermatology* 138 (6): 771–74.

Bulliard, J. 2000. Site specific risk of cutaneous malignant melanoma and pattern exposure in New Zealand. *International Journal of Cancer* 85 (5): 627–32.

Byrd, K., D. Wilson, S. Hoyler, and G. Peck. 2004. Advanced presentation of melanoma in African Americans. *Journal of the American Academy of Dermatology* 50 (1): 21–24, 142–43.

CDC. *See* Centers for Disease Control.

Cancer Council Australia. 2002. Sun protection and babies. *Position Statement,* www.cancer.org.au.

———. 2003. Vitamin D. *Position Statement,* www.cancer. org.au.

Cancer Council New South Wales. 2002. Call for urgent regulation of sun-bed industry. *Media Releases* 923, February 7.

Carter, R., R. Marks, and D. Hill. 1999. Could a national skin cancer primary prevention campaign in Australia be worthwhile? An economic perspective. *Health Promotion International* 14 (1): 73–82.

Centers for Disease Control. 1998. Sun protection behaviors used by adults for children. *Morbidity and Mortality Weekly Report* 47 (23): 480–82.

———. 2004. Preventing America's most common cancer. *Skin Cancer Fact Sheet,* http://www.cdc.gov/cancer/nscpep/skinpdfs/about2004.pdf

Conlan, K. 2003. The sun, another construction site hazard. *The Skin Cancer Foundation Journal* 21:24–26.

Cooke, K., and J. Fraser. 1985. Migration and death from malignant melanoma. *International Journal of Cancer* 36:175–78.

Coppertone. 2002. A history of Coppertone innovations. http://www.coppertone.ca/english/solar/sun_care_history.cfm

Dellavalle, R., E. Parker, N. Cernsonsky, E. Hester, B. Hemme, D. Brukhardt, S. Chen, and L. Shilling. 2003. Youth access laws: In the dark at the tanning parlor. *Archives of Dermatology* 139:443–48, 520–24.

Diffey, B., and J. Cheeseman. 1992. Sun protection with hats. *British Journal of Dermatology* 127:10–12.

Elwood, J. 1992. Melanoma and sun exposure: Contrasts between intermittent and chronic exposure. *World Journal of Surgery* 16 (2): 157–65.

FDA. *See* Food and Drug Administration.

Feldman, S., A. Liguori, M. Kucenin, S. Rapp, A. Fleicher, W. Lang, and M. Kaur. 2004. Ultraviolet exposure is a reinforcing stimulus in frequent indoor tanners. *Journal of the American Academy of Dermatology* 51:45–51.

Food and Drug Administration. 2004. FDA approves new use of drug to treat superficial basal cell carcinoma, a type of skin cancer. *FDA News* (Press Release) PO4-66.

Fraser, P., W. Ding, M. Mohseni, E. Treadwell, M. Dooley, E. St. Clair, G. Gilkeson, and G. Cooper. 2003. Glutathione S-transferase M null homozygosity and risk of systemic lupus erythematosus associated with sun exposure: A possible gene-environment interaction for autoimmunity. *Journal of Rheumatology* 30 (2): 276–82.

Gambichler, T., A. Avermaete, A. Bader, P. Altmeyer, and K. Hoffman. 2001. Ultraviolet protection by summer textiles. Ultraviolet transmission measurements verified by determination of the minimal erythema dose with solar-simulated radiation. *British Journal of Dermatology* 144 (3): 449–50.

Gartner, L., and F. Greer. 2003. Prevention of rickets and Vitamin D deficiency: New guidelines for vitamin D intake. *Pediatrics* 111 (4): 908–10.

Geller, A., G. Colditz, S. Oliveria, K. Emmons, C. Jorgenson, G. Aweh, and L. Frazier. 2002. Use of sunscreen, sunburning rates, and tanning bed use among more than 10,000 U.S. children and adolescents. *Pediatrics* 109 (6): 1009–14.

Geller, A., Z. Zhang, A. Sober, A. Halpern, M. Weinstock, S. Daniels, D. Miller, M. Demierre, D. Brooks, and B. Gilchrest. 2003. The first 15 years of the American Academy of Dermatology Skin Cancer Screening Programs: 1985–1999. *Journal of the American Academy of Dermatology* 48 (1): 34–41.

Gies, P., C. Roy, and G. Elliot. 1990. A proposed UVR protection factor for sunglasses. *Clinical and Experimental Optometry* 73 (6): 184–89.

Gies, P., C. Roy, S. Toomey, and A. McLennan. 1998. Protection against solar ultraviolet radiation. *Mutation Research* 422:15–22.

Gies, P., C. Roy, S. Toomey, and D. Tomlinson. 1999. Ambient solar UVR, personal exposure, and protection. *Journal of Epidemiology* 9 (6): 115–22.

Gies, P., C. Roy, and W. Zongli. 1992. Ultraviolet radiation protection factors for clear and tinted automobile windscreens. *Radiation Protection in Australia* 10 (4): 91–94.

Gies, P., and J. Wright. 2003. Measured solar ultraviolet radiation exposure of outdoor workers in Queensland in the building construction industry. *Photochemistry and Photobiology* 78 (4): 342–48.

Godar, D. 2001. UV doses of american children and adolescents. *Photochemistry and Photobiology* 74 (6): 787–93.

Godar, D., F. Urbach, F. Gasparro, and J. van der Leun. 2003. UV doses of young adults. *Photochemistry and Photobiology* 77 (4): 453–57.

Godar, D., S. Wengraitis, J. Shreffler, and D. Sliney. 2001. UV doses of Americans. *Photochemistry and Photobiology* 73 (6): 621–29.

Halpern, A., and L. Kopp. 2004. Awareness, knowledge, and attitudes to nonmelanoma skin cancer and actinic keratoses among the general public. *International Journal of Dermatology* online, doi:10.111/j.1365-4632.2004.02090.x

Hunter Douglas Windows. 2004. Living in style. www.hunterdouglas.com/living_in_style.jsp (accessed June 12, 2004).

Hurwitz, S. 1988. The sun and sunscreen protection: Recommendations for children. *Journal of Dermatological Surgical Oncology* 14 (6): 657–60.

ILSF. *See* International Life Saving Federation.

International Life Saving Federation. 2004. Statements on sun dangers for lifeguards. *Medical Position Statements*, www.ilsf.org.

Jemal, A., S. Deveso, P. Hartge, and M. Tucker. 2001. Recent trends in cutaneous melanoma incidence among whites in the United States. *Journal of the National Cancer Institute* 93 (9): 678–83.

Johnson, K., L. Davy, T. Boyett, L. Weathers, and R. Roetzheim. 2001. Sun protection practices in children and the increase in skin cancers. *Archives of Pediatrics and Adolescent Medicine* 155:891–96.

Kenet, B., and P. Lawler. 1998. *Saving Your Skin: Prevention, Early Detection, and Treatment of Melanoma and Other Skin Cancers.* New York: Four Walls Eight Windows.

Kirkwood, J., M. Strawderman, M. Ernstoff, T. Smith, E. Borden, and R. Blum. 1996. Interferon alfa-2b adjuvant therapy of high risk resected cutaneous melanoma: The Eastern Cooperative Oncology Group trial. *Journal of Clinical Oncology* 14:7–17.

Koh, H., D. Miller, A. Geller, R. Clapp, M. Mercer, and R. Lew. 1992. Who discovers melanoma? Patterns from a population based survey. *Journal of the American Academy of Dermatology* 26:914–19.

Kubler, V. 1999. Interior fashion focus: Solar control—The intelligent choice. *Draperies and Window Coverings Magazine,* November. www.dwc designet.com/DWC/Nov'99/solar.html.

Levine, H. 2004. A killer tan. Burning issue: Are UV rays in tanning beds really safe? *Prevention Magazine,* May, 156–61, 195–98, 202.

Lupus Foundation. 2004. Statistics about lupus. www.lupus.org.

Lupus UK. 2004. Lupus fact sheet. www.lupusuk.com

Mack, T., and B. Floderus. 1991. Malignant melanoma risk by nativity, place of residence at diagnosis, age at migration. *Cancer Causes and Control* 2 (6): 401–11.

MarketResearch.com. 2002. *Drugs and Cosmetics for Aging Boomers: A Surging Market.* Publication ID no. WA763975.

Marks, R. 1996. The use of sunscreen in the prevention of skin cancer. *Cancer Forum* 20:211–15.

Masci, P., and E. Borden. 2002. Malignant melanoma: Treatments emerging but early detection is still key. *Cleveland Clinic Journal of Medicine* 69 (7): 529–45.

Mathers, C., R. Penm, R. Sanson-Fisher, and E. Campbell. 1998. Health system costs of cancer in Australia, 1993–94. Canberra. *AIHW and the National Cancer Control Initiative* 4:1–42.

Meadows, M. 2002. Saving your sight: Early detection is critical. *FDA Consumer Magazine* 36 (2): 22–28.

Melanoma Center. 2004. Skin cancer screenings. *Prevention,* http://www.mel anomacenter.org/prevention/screenings.html.

Mintel Market Researchers. 2001. The sun care market. *U.S. Consumer Intelligence,* May, 26.

NCI. *See* National Cancer Institute.

NMSS. *See* National Multiple Sclerosis Society.

NOAH. *See* National Organization for Albinism and Hypopigmentation.

NZDS. *See* New Zealand Dermatological Society.

National Cancer Institute. 2003a. Eating hints for cancer patients: Before, during, and after treatment. *Cancer Topics,* www.nci.nih.gov/cancertopics/ eatinghints.

National Eye Institute. 2004. Age-related macular degeneration: What you should know. http://www.nei.nih.gov/health/maculardegen/armd_facts.asp.

National Multiple Sclerosis Society. 2004. Who gets MS? *About MS,* www.nationalmssociety.org.

National Organization for Albinism and Hypopigmentation. 2002. What is albinism? www.albinism.org.

New Zealand Dermatological Society. 2004. Global solar ultraviolet index. *DermNetNZ,* http://www.dermnetnz.org/site-age-specific/UV-index.html

Odom, R. 2004. Actinic keratoses today. *The Skin Cancer Foundation Journal* 22:44–45, 88.

Pathak, M. 1999. What sunscreen can and cannot do. *The Melanoma Letter* 17 (2).

———. 2002. What sunscreen can and cannot do. *The Skin Cancer Foundation Journal* 20:49–52.

Pathak, M., K. Jimbow, and T. Fitzpatrick. 1976. Sunlight and melanin pigmentation. In *Photochemical and Photobiologic Reviews,* edited by K. Smith. Vol. 1. New York: Plenum.

Patient UK. 2004. Melanoma. *Leaflets,* www.patient.co.uk/showdoc/270 00650.

Pfahlberg, A., F. Kolmel, and O. Gefeller for the Febim Study Group. 2001. Timing of excessive ultraviolet radiation and melanoma: Epidemiology does not support the existence of a critical period of high susceptibility to solar ultraviolet radiation induced melanoma. *British Journal of Dermatology* 144 (3): 471–76.

Poole, C. M., and D. Guerry. 1998. *Melanoma: Prevention, Detection, and Treatment.* New Haven, Conn.: Yale University Press.

Population Reference Bureau. 2000. The aging of the United States, 1999–2025. *Ameristat,* August, 1–3.

Pouliot, J. S. 2003. Tanning troubles: Lured by aggressive marketing, young adults are flocking to tanning salons—and being exposed to skin cancer dangers once only found at the beach. *Better Homes and Gardens,* May, 81–87.

Reid, C. 1996. Chemical photosensitivity another reason to be careful in the sun. *FDA Consumer Magazine,* May. http://www.fda.gov/fdac/features/496_sun.html

SCF. *See* The Skin Cancer Foundation.

SEER. *See* Surveillance, Epidemiology, and End Results.

Scotto, J. 1986. Nonmelanoma skin cancer—UVB effects. In *Stratospheric Ozone,* volume 2 of *Effects of Changes in Stratospheric Ozone and Global Climate,* edited by J. Titus. Proceedings of the United Nations Environment Program/Environmental Protection Agency International Conference on Health and Environmental Effects of Ozone Modification and Climate Change. Washington, D.C.: U.S. Environmental Protection Agency.

Sekula-Gibbs, S. 2004. Tanning: Harsh reality vs. fiction. *The Skin Cancer Foundation Journal* 22:34–38.

Sjögren's Syndrome Foundation. 2004. What is Sjögren's syndrome? *About Sjögren's Syndrome,* www.sjogrens.org/syndrome.

The Skin Cancer Foundation. 2001. If you can spot it, you can stop it. *How to Spot Skin Cancer,* www.skincancer.org/self-exam/spot_skin_cancer.php

———. 2002. Old brown eyes. *Sun and Skin News* 19 (4): 4.

———. 2003a. New warning to older black women: Watch out for skin cancers on the legs. *Sun and Skin News* 20 (1): 4.

———. 2003b. Skin cancer: A concern for all ages. *Older Adults,* www.skincancer.org/older/index.php.

————. 2003c. The newest cancer epidemic is an eye opener. *News,* www.skincancer.org/news/031110-epidemic.php.

————. 2004a. About basal cell carcinoma. *Public Information Materials,* www.skincancer.org/basal/index.php.

————. 2004b. About melanoma. *Public Information Materials,* www.skincancer.org/melanoma/index.php.

————. 2005. *Understanding Melanoma: What You Need to Know.* 2nd ed. New York: The Skin Cancer Foundation.

Sliney, D. 1986. Physical factors in cataractogenesis: Ambient ultraviolet radiation and temperature. *Investigative Ophthalmology and Visual Science* 27:781–90.

Stern, R., M. Weinstein, and S. Baker. 1986. Risk reduction for non-melanoma skin cancer with childhood sunscreen use. *Archives of Dermatology* 122:537–45. Cited in Godar, D., F. Urbach, F. Gasparro, and J. van der Leun. 2003. UV doses of young adults. *Photochemistry and Photobiology* 77 (4): 453–57.

Stokes, R., and B. Diffey. 1997. How well are sunscreen users protected? *Photodermatology, Photoimmunology & Photomedicine* 13:186–88.

Surveillance, Epidemiology, and End Results. 2001. SEER Program Public Use Data (1973–1998), NCI, DCCPS, Cancer Surveillance Research Program, Cancer Statistics Branch.

Taylor, H., S. West, F. Rosenthal, B. Munoz, H. Newland, H. Abbey, and E. Emmett. 1988. Effect of ultraviolet radiation on cataract formation. *New England Journal of Medicine* 319 (22): 1429–33.

Taylor, S., and Z. Rahman. 2001. Melanoma in the African American population. *The Melanoma Letter* 19:2.

Tsao, H., G. Rogers, and A. Sober. 1998. An estimate of the annual direct cost of treating cutaneous melanoma. *Journal of the American Academy of Dermatology* 38:669–80.

Tucker, M., E. Halpern, P. Holly, R. Elder, D. Sagebiel, D. Guerry IV, and W. Clark Jr. 1997. Clinically recognized dysplastic nevi. A central risk factor for cutaneous melanoma. *Journal of the American Medical Association* 277(18):1439–44.

USDHHS, FDA, [and?] CDRH. *See* United States Department of Health and Human Services, Food and Drug Administration, [and?] Center for Devices and Radiological Health.

United States Department of Health and Human Services, Food and Drug Administration, Center for Devices and Radiological Health. 1998. Guidance document for nonprescription sunglasses: Introduction. *CDRH Facts on Demand #2208,* http://www.fda.gov/cdrh/ode/90.html.

Wong, J., R. Airey, and R. Fleming. 1996. Annual reduction of solar UV exposure to the facial area of outdoor workers in Southeast Queensland by wearing a hat. *Photodermatology, Photoimmunology & Photomedicine* 12:131–35.

Wooley, T., P. Buettner, and J. Lowe. 2002. Sun-related behaviors of outdoor working men with a history of nonmelanoma skin cancer. *Journal of Occupational and Environmental Medicine* 44 (9): 847–54.

Wright, M., S. Wright, and F. Wagner. 2001. Mechanisms of sunscreen failure. *Journal of the American Academy of Dermatology* 44 (5): 781–84.

XPS. *See* Xeroderma Pigmentosum Society.

Xeroderma Pigmentosum Society. 2004. About XP. http://www.xps.org/xp.htm

Younan, C., P. Mitchell, R. Cumming, E. Rochtchina, and J. Wang. 2002. Iris color and incident ca taract and cataract surgery: The Blue Mountain Eye Study. *American Journal of Ophthalmology* 134 (2): 273–74.

Mary Mills Barrow and John F. Barrow are cofounders of Coolibar, a company specializing in sun protective products and clothing. The Skin Cancer Foundation has recognized the Barrows as experts in the field of sun protection: Coolibar is the only sun protection clothing company recommended by the foundation.

For more information about Coolibar, please visit **www.coolibar.com.**

Mary Mills Barrow has worked in several New York publishing houses and as an editor for McKinsey & Co, Inc., an international management-consulting firm. She works as a communications consultant for Coolibar. She lived in Australia for a decade, learning firsthand the importance of sun protection for adults and children.

John Barrow has an extensive background in business and publishing. He holds a master's degree in business administration from Harvard University. Mr. Barrow is currently the President of Coolibar. He grew up in Sydney, Australia.

Foreword writer **Albert Rosenthal, MD,** is clinical professor of dermatology at Drexel University's Hahnemann Medical College

Some Other
New Harbinger Titles

Eating Mindfully, Item 3503, $13.95

Living with RSDS, Item 3554 $16.95

The Ten Hidden Barriers to Weight Loss, Item 3244 $11.95

The Sjogren's Syndrome Survival Guide, Item 3562 $15.95

Stop Feeling Tired, Item 3139 $14.95

Responsible Drinking, Item 2949 $18.95

The Mitral Valve Prolapse/Dysautonomia Survival Guide, Item 3031 $14.95

Stop Worrying Abour Your Health, Item 285X $14.95

The Vulvodynia Survival Guide, Item 2914 $15.95

The Multifidus Back Pain Solution, Item 2787 $12.95

Move Your Body, Tone Your Mood, Item 2752 $17.95

The Chronic Illness Workbook, Item 2647 $16.95

Coping with Crohn's Disease, Item 2655 $15.95

The Woman's Book of Sleep, Item 2493 $14.95

The Trigger Point Therapy Workbook, Item 2507 $19.95

Fibromyalgia and Chronic Myofascial Pain Syndrome, second edition, Item 2388 $19.95

Kill the Craving, Item 237X $18.95

Rosacea, Item 2248 $13.95

Thinking Pregnant, Item 2302 $13.95

Shy Bladder Syndrome, Item 2272 $13.95

Help for Hairpullers, Item 2329 $13.95

Coping with Chronic Fatigue Syndrome, Item 0199 $13.95

Call **toll free, 1-800-748-6273,** or log on to our online bookstore at **www.newharbinger.com** to order. Have your Visa or Mastercard number ready. Or send a check for the titles you want to New Harbinger Publications, Inc., 5674 Shattuck Ave., Oakland, CA 94609. Include $4.50 for the first book and 75¢ for each additional book, to cover shipping and handling. (California residents please include appropriate sales tax.) Allow two to five weeks for delivery.

Prices subject to change without notice.